JUST MOVE!

A NEW APPROACH TO FITNESS AFTER **50**

JUST MOVE!

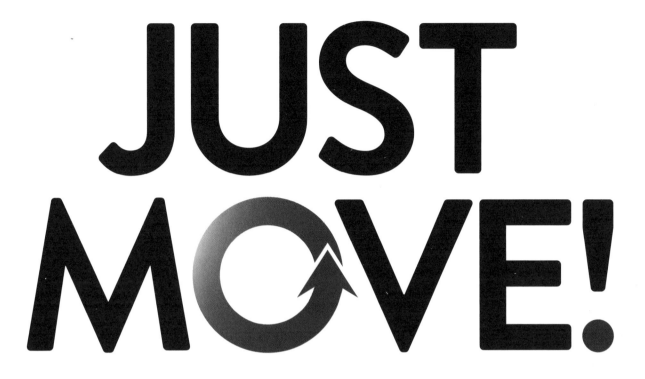

A NEW APPROACH TO FITNESS AFTER 50

James P. Owen

WITH

BRIGITTE LeBLANC

DESIGN **NITA ALVAREZ**

ILLUSTRATION **DAVID PREISS**

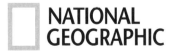 NATIONAL GEOGRAPHIC

WASHINGTON, D.C.

Since 1888, the National Geographic Society has funded more than 12,000 research, exploration, and preservation projects around the world. National Geographic Partners distributes a portion of the funds it receives from your purchase to National Geographic Society to support programs including the conservation of animals and their habitats.

National Geographic Partners
1145 17th Street NW
Washington, DC 20036-4688 USA

Become a member of National Geographic and activate your benefits today at natgeo.com/jointoday.

For information about special discounts for bulk purchases, please contact National Geographic Books Special Sales: specialsales@natgeo.com

For rights or permissions inquiries, please contact National Geographic Books Subsidiary Rights: bookrights@natgeo.com

Important Note to Readers

This book is for educational purposes and is not intended as medical or other professional advice to the individual reader. You should not use the information contained in this book as a substitute for the advice of a licensed health care professional. You should consult a licensed health care professional before beginning an exercise program. To the best of our knowledge, the information provided is accurate at the time of its publication.

The author and publisher disclaim any liability whatsoever with respect to any loss, injury, or damage arising directly or indirectly from the use of this book.

ISBN: 978-1-4262-1865-1
Printed in the United States of America
17/QGT-LSCML/1

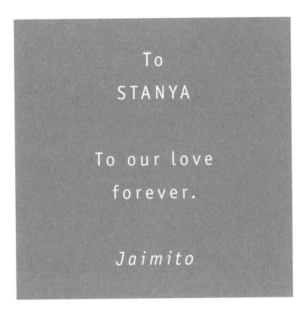

To
STANYA

To our love
forever.

Jaimito

T A B L E   O F

USING THIS BOOK

*This is one fitness guide that puts **you** in charge. It is written specifically for people north of 50, by a former couch potato who's decidedly within that demographic.*

It aims to be inspiring, even empowering, while giving you just enough knowledge to create your own exercise program—fitness basics you need to know, with no confusing buzzwords or information overload.

It's also realistic. I'm not promising quick, dramatic results. But you can become measurably more fit over time if you consistently devote one hour a day to following a program along the lines I've outlined.

The book gives you a flexible, step-by-step program you can tailor to your needs and preferences.

Finally, it's modular, so you can read it any way you want. You can dip in and out of chapters, skim for the most relevant nuggets, or revisit chapters whenever you want a reminder or a fresh shot of motivation.

CONTENTS

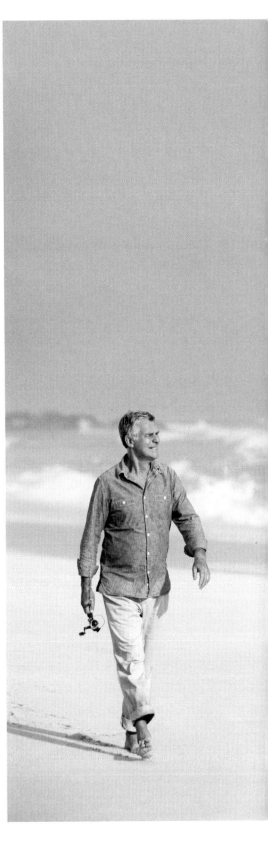

Foreword

JUST MOVE! This call to action has been espoused by public health advocates, health care practitioners, and fitness experts for years. Yet exercise, considered by many medical scientists to be the magic bullet for good health, is underappreciated and underutilized as a means of achieving and sustaining a healthy life, particularly in later years. While the public health message recommending a minimum of 30 minutes of aerobic exercise on five or more days of the week is widely known, there is less appreciation that this message is targeting those who need it most—the sedentary couch potatoes among us. There is tremendous health benefit to be gained by leaving their ranks and becoming a regular exerciser. *Just Move!* takes this message a step further. In this book, author Jim Owen describes his personal voyage to functional fitness and the sensibly crafted program he developed to achieve and maintain it.

Functional fitness is an especially important concept for aging adults, who can use a well-rounded exercise program to offset age-related decline in physical capabilities. While that decline is due partly to normal aging, much is also due to physical deconditioning and disuse. The good news is that deconditioning and disuse are reversible with exercise—and age doesn't matter! Even for those well into their nineties, starting to exercise will result in substantial benefits. This is true even—and especially—if you suffer from common chronic illnesses such as diabetes, heart disease, arthritis, or high blood pressure. Functional fitness combines cardio/endurance exercise with strengthening, flexibility, balance, and functional exercises, all aimed at making it easy to manage daily physical tasks. As a side benefit, functional fitness will also contribute to optimal management of many chronic illnesses.

The book you hold in your hand is an ideal guide for those who want to be more fit but aren't sure how or whether they can achieve that goal. It is also useful for those who are already exercising and want to get more results from their efforts. *Just Move!* can serve as an encouraging and informed friend, clearly pointing to ideas for, and describing the benefits of, taking that first, tenth, and hundredth step to making functional fitness a priority. At age 70, plagued by back pain, Jim Owen began his quest for health. He decided that his visits to the gym would not be about how much weight he could lift or lose, but about how he could become functionally fit. Following an exercise routine based on functional fitness will likewise allow you to accomplish your everyday activities with ease, from climbing stairs to lifting groceries, while maximizing your independence in late life. In short, it will help you live the life you want.

Just Move! will walk you through a progressive approach to functional fitness with an abundance of practical pointers and meaningful insights. This book is highly motivating with lots of easy-to-follow tips to help make your voyage engaging and feasible. Take it to heart and make functional fitness an important part of every day for the rest of your life. You are worth it!

DR. MIRIAM C. MOREY

Professor of Geriatric Medicine
Duke University School of Medicine

Co-Director, Duke Claude D. Pepper
Older Americans Independence Center

Dr. Miriam C. Morey is one of the leading experts in aging-related functional fitness in the United States. She has more than 30 years of experience in the field of geriatric fitness and is also the associate director of research of the Geriatric Research, Education and Clinical Center of the Durham Veterans Affairs Medical Center in North Carolina. She directs a clinical exercise program for older veterans, called Gerofit, which is being nationally disseminated at selected VA medical centers around the country. In her spare time she enjoys playing competitive tennis.

AN IDEAL GUIDE FOR THOSE WHO WANT TO BE MORE FIT BUT AREN'T SURE HOW OR WHETHER THEY CAN ACHIEVE THAT GOAL.

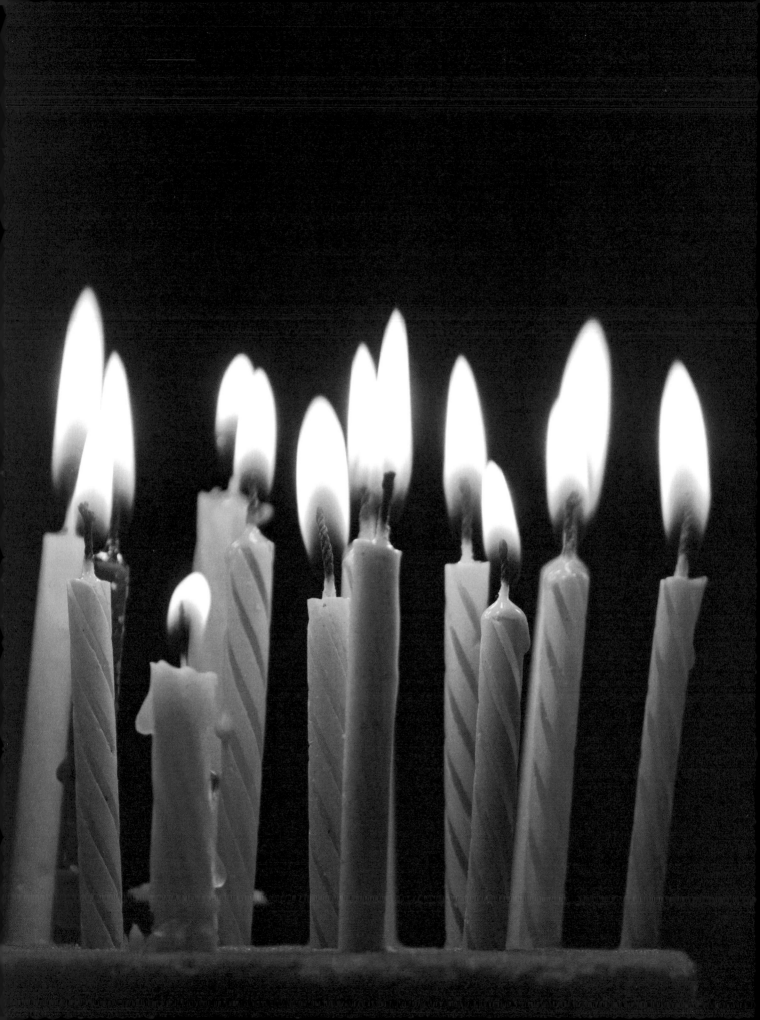

Fit at 50, 60, 70?
It's Never Too Late

THE FACT that you've picked up this book says a couple of things about you. Given the title on the cover, I'm guessing you're somewhere in the age bracket when decades of physical wear and tear usually start having some effects, even if you've always been as healthy as the proverbial horse.

And you're probably thinking that doing more to get or stay fit would be a good idea. If you're not already doing some kind of exercise at least four or five days a week and addressing the multiple dimensions of fitness in the process—including strength, conditioning, flexibility, and balance—I'd say you're absolutely right!

Having made it this far, you've already benefited from some combination of good genes, good circumstances, and good luck. Statistically speaking, someone who reaches the age of 70 can now expect to be around for his or her 85th birthday—and that's just the average.

Depending on your age and condition, you might have another 20, 25, 30, or even more years on this planet. Longevity in developed nations generally has been increasing at the rate of three months a year for decades. Who knows what coming medical breakthroughs might further accelerate those gains? At research institutions across the country, scientists are busy working to decipher the mechanisms of the aging process and find new ways of extending human life span and "health span"—the length of time we stay healthy and fully functional. It may not be that long before turning 100 is no longer exceptional.

Now is the time to think about what you want the next chapter of your life to be like. If you're physically out of shape—or even a certified couch potato, like I used to be—you might assume it's all downhill from here in any case. When a steep flight of stairs starts to feel like Mount Kilimanjaro, can a cane or walker be far behind? Maybe you're simply in denial, figuring it's too late to do anything about it, anyway.

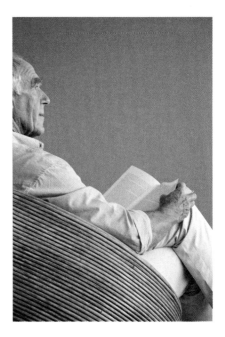

NOW IS THE TIME TO THINK ABOUT WHAT YOU WANT THE NEXT CHAPTER OF YOUR LIFE TO BE LIKE.

> EXERCISE IS THE BEST TOOL WE HAVE AGAINST AGING.
> IF IT WERE A DRUG, IT WOULD BE PRESCRIBED FOR EVERYBODY.
>
> DR. GORDON LITHGOW
> *Geneticist,* Buck Institute for Research on Aging

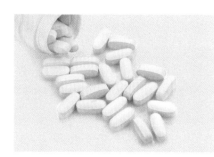

Either way, my message is the same. To borrow a phrase from Ira Gershwin, it ain't necessarily so.

In the last 20 years scientists have learned there's a lot more we can do to slow the pace of aging than was formerly thought. But physical activity is still the closest thing there is to a magic bullet. "Exercise is the best tool we have against aging," says Dr. Gordon Lithgow, a geneticist at the Buck Institute for Research on Aging in northern California. "If it were a drug, it would be prescribed for everybody."

What's more, studies show that even a moderate amount of exercise can go a long way toward improving your physical functioning and maintaining your quality of life, even if you don't start until later in life. A whole fitness culture is beginning to blossom around the baby boomer generation, with a growing number of trainers, exercise classes, and gyms aimed specifically at that demographic. Experts agree that as long as you retain some level of mobility, it's never too late to become more fit.

So it's interesting to me that gray hair is still so rarely seen in fitness books and magazines. As you browse those bookstore shelves, you see plenty of covers breathlessly promising that in a matter of weeks, you, too, can be leaner, healthier, and sexier, just like the sleek and well-muscled 20- or 30-somethings in the photographs.

This is not that kind of book.

You'll also see more serious volumes, some of them aimed at an "older" population of 40- or 50-year-olds. Often authored by people with M.D.'s, Ph.D.'s, or both, they typically walk you through a crash course on exercise physiology, and then give you enough exercises for a whole squadron of Royal Canadian Mounties.

This is not that kind of book, either.

Just to be clear, I'm not a doctor, a trainer, a celebrity endorser of the newest exercise fad, or a fitness guru of any kind. I'm a reformed couch potato in my seventies who wants to share the lessons I've learned along the way as well as the perspectives and tips I've gleaned from others.

What I've endeavored to write is the book I wish I'd had at the beginning of my fitness journey—one with as much inspiration as information. One that clearly lays out a flexible plan anyone can follow. A book that strips things down to the essentials you really need to know, and not much more. I hope I can save you a lot of the effort I spent sorting through all the hype and conflicting advice out there.

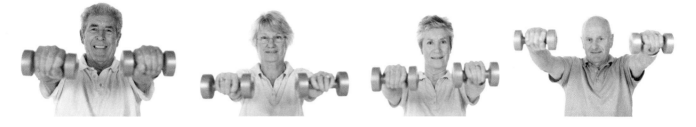

To be honest, if someone had told me six years ago that I'd be authoring a book about fitness, I'd have laughed out loud. As I approached my 70th birthday, I was hurting all over. Years of sitting at a desk and all too frequent airplane trips had taken their toll. My lower back was killing me, to the point where I was getting epidural injections just to make the pain bearable. I had two bad knees, the legacy of a running regimen I'd impulsively started in my fifties with no clue how to keep from getting injured. My right rotator cuff was in bad shape from improperly hauling heavy luggage. My shoulders were rounded and I was so stooped I couldn't even stand up straight.

My wake-up call came on the very day I turned 70, when I saw a video of me shuffling up to a podium to give a speech. I was shocked! What happened to the energy and confidence I'd had all my life? Was my physique really that slack? Somehow I had turned into the poster child for looming old age.

I knew I had to do something—and it had to be radically different than my haphazard attempts at fitness in the past. Like a lot of guys, I'd always associated being fit with bulging muscles. Though I tried my hand at sports in high school, and managed to bulk up to 205 pounds, I was still slow and awkward. Most games I spent warming the bench. By the time I was in college, I'd given up on organized sports. And once I graduated, I was so preoccupied with building a career that physical fitness didn't even cross my mind. For some 30 years I had no exercise program at all.

Then came my second bout of trying to get in shape. Your typical weekend warrior, I started running the hills around my house on my days off, figuring I'd better hit it hard to make up for all my hours in a chair. I also set up a gym at home and hired someone to help me train. He had me bench-pressing 200 pounds when I felt a searing pain shoot down my spine. He told me I should "work through" the pain, but I couldn't do it. My back, my knees, my whole body rebelled.

After sitting around for a year as my waistband grew tighter, I spent a week at Canyon Ranch in Tucson, learning how to eat right and control my weight. I was too dispirited even to attempt another exercise program.

A WHOLE FITNESS CULTURE IS BEGINNING TO BLOSSOM AROUND THE BABY BOOMER GENERATION.

GETTING FIT IS NOWHERE NEAR AS HARD AS DEALING WITH THE INFIRMITIES OF OLD AGE.

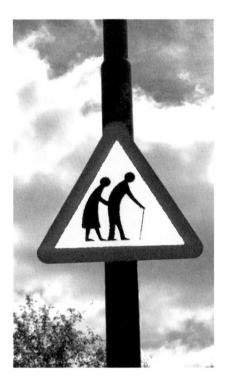

I succeeded in getting down to 180 pounds, a good number for my six-foot-one-inch frame. The trouble was, I looked haggard and felt stiff and weak. While shedding fat, I'd also lost much of what little muscle mass had remained. It was as plain as day that diet alone wasn't enough to get my body into shape.

This time would be different, I vowed. In my encore career as an author and speaker, I'd just written a book called *The Try*, about people who were inspiring in the way they set a goal, pursued it unflaggingly, and gave their all to that one thing they passionately wanted to do. As I slid into my seventies, I knew staving off old age was something I could be passionate about! And now, in between traveling to speaking engagements around the country, I could finally take as much time as I needed to get in shape.

I dove into a stack of fitness magazines, trying to sift practical tips from the confusing torrent of exhortations ("get rock-hard abs in 30 days!") and pumping-iron jargon ("start with a single-arm clean and press"). There was plenty of advice out there, but it was a mixed bag, and a good bit of it seemed dubious even to a novice like me. As I read "see how many dead lifts you can do in 60 seconds," I could already picture myself on my way to the ER.

The critical first step, I realized, was getting clear on what I wanted to accomplish. I was determined not to repeat my mistakes of the past. For starters, I banished any lingering mental images of myself with rippling muscles. Ego and vanity weren't going to derail me.

I'd figured out that functional fitness was what I really needed. Yes, I wanted to gain enough strength to carry my suitcase or move a box from the closet without throwing out my back. But above all, I wanted to learn how to move. My biggest goal was to be able to carry on the ordinary activities of life without hurting myself or being hobbled by stiffness and pain. I imagined myself in ten years, easily striding up a stairway or dipping down into a deep squat to pick up something dropped on the floor. Staying mobile, active, and energetic—that was the future I wanted.

The next step was finding the right person to guide me. A good trainer would help me get over the intimidation I felt when walking into a gym. Most of all, I needed someone knowledgeable to work with me over the long haul—someone with the expertise to know what I should do, given my physical limitations, and the patience to show me how to do it without hurting myself.

Luckily for me, I now live in Austin, and fitness is as big a part of that city's culture as indie music and barbecue. My wife and I moved in to a high-rise building partly because it had its own gym. Based on some research and trusted referrals, I then hired an experienced and accredited personal trainer, Scott Gassner. Unlike some of the other trainers I interviewed, Scottie had worked with a number of older clients with issues similar to mine. He asked me a lot of insightful questions, and I liked his clear, practical approach. He himself was clearly fit, but he was by no means a muscle-bound hulk like some of the bodybuilding zealots I'd encountered.

Just knowing I'd have Scottie in my corner boosted my confidence level, though that didn't last long. My first workout with him was downright embarrassing. I couldn't do a single push-up correctly! But we both hung in there, and with Scottie's help I began mastering some basic moves. We worked together for one hour at a time, three times a week, adding exercises and repetitions little by little. I also started paying attention to the ways I was moving outside the gym, applying what Scottie was teaching me about good form and body mechanics.

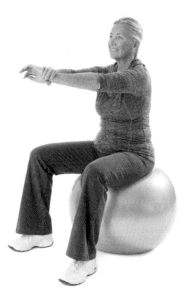

IT'S NOT ABOUT
HAVING TIME...
IT'S ABOUT
MAKING TIME.

Week by week, each small increment of progress led me to the next. I could see myself slowly becoming stronger and more solid. Thanks to all the core-strengthening work we were doing, my back problems virtually disappeared. I was enjoying my daily walks and spent more time stretching. And I started to see my improvements in the gym carrying over into the rest of my life. Getting in and out of the car, carrying groceries, even just moving from place to place—as the months went by, I found myself able to do all these things with more ease and fluidity than I'd felt in years.

Of course, human progress is never a straight line, and I've certainly run into my share of hurdles along the way. I wanted my workouts to be challenging, and they are. There have been times when I've pushed myself right up to my limits. I can't help feeling disheartened when I feel a twinge of pain after making a wrong move. And I'm still bedeviled by a stubborn tightness in my hips and ankles, alleviated only by regular sessions of yoga and Pilates. But I'm going to keep working on it as long as I am able.

What keeps me motivated is a stark reality: Getting fit is nowhere near as hard as dealing with the infirmities of old age.

It's one thing to be in your sixties or seventies and wish you'd started an exercise program 20 years ago. You can still gain physical stamina and function, even if you have arthritis, weigh more than you'd like, or have other barriers to overcome. It's another thing to be in your eighties or nineties, and so frail or wracked with pain that every step takes all the effort you can muster. Who doesn't want to avoid that by any means possible?

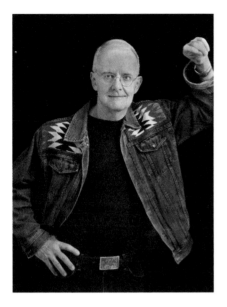

SPENDING AN
HOUR A DAY ON
FITNESS HAS BEEN
THE BEST INVESTMENT
I EVER MADE.

At the same time, nobody's saying you have to turn into Superman or Wonder Woman to become more fit than you are now. Maybe you've always been strong, or you're the kind of person who likes to push hard and keep raising the bar. Or maybe you'd rather have a less demanding, lower-key program aimed at maintaining the level of fitness you have now. Or maybe you're somewhere in between.

Whatever your goals and preferences, this book is designed to help you pursue the fitness program that works for you, taking it one step at a time. While it's true that I'm a strong advocate of working out at a gym with a skilled trainer, you may not prefer or be able to go that route. You can still benefit from the program I've outlined. Similarly, if you do the "getting started" program for three months and decide that activity level is enough for you, that's fine. Anything you do to be active is all to the good. The important thing is to get moving!

As I write this, I'm well past my 75th birthday, and I feel great! In fact, my doctor was startled with my test results at my last checkup: a low resting heart rate, rapid recovery rate after exertion, normal blood pressure, and a significant drop in my LDL cholesterol (the "bad" one). What's more, I can now do a lot of things I couldn't when I was 30. After working hard at it for several years, I've gone from being unable to do a single proper push-up to doing 50. I'm now in the best shape of my life.

Best of all, getting fit has transformed my relationship with my body. In the beginning I worked out because I felt I had to. Now I work out because I *want* to. It's something I genuinely enjoy and look forward to. Fitness has become my most satisfying hobby.

After all these years, I've finally escaped the sedentary lifestyle and found my inner athlete. My friends say I look younger and more vigorous, which is always gratifying to hear. But that's not what it's all about. What really makes me proud is knowing I've taken charge of my future. I've done what's in my power to make my life a long and healthy one. If this book can help even a few people move in the same direction, it will be the best legacy I could have.

JIM OWEN
Austin, Texas

PART ONE

WHAT EVERYONE
OVER 50
SHOULD KNOW

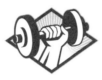

Aging Sooner, or Later—Which Will It Be?

❖

How to Succeed at Fitness

❖

Functional Fitness—What It Means, Why You Need It

❖

5 Facets of Functional Fitness

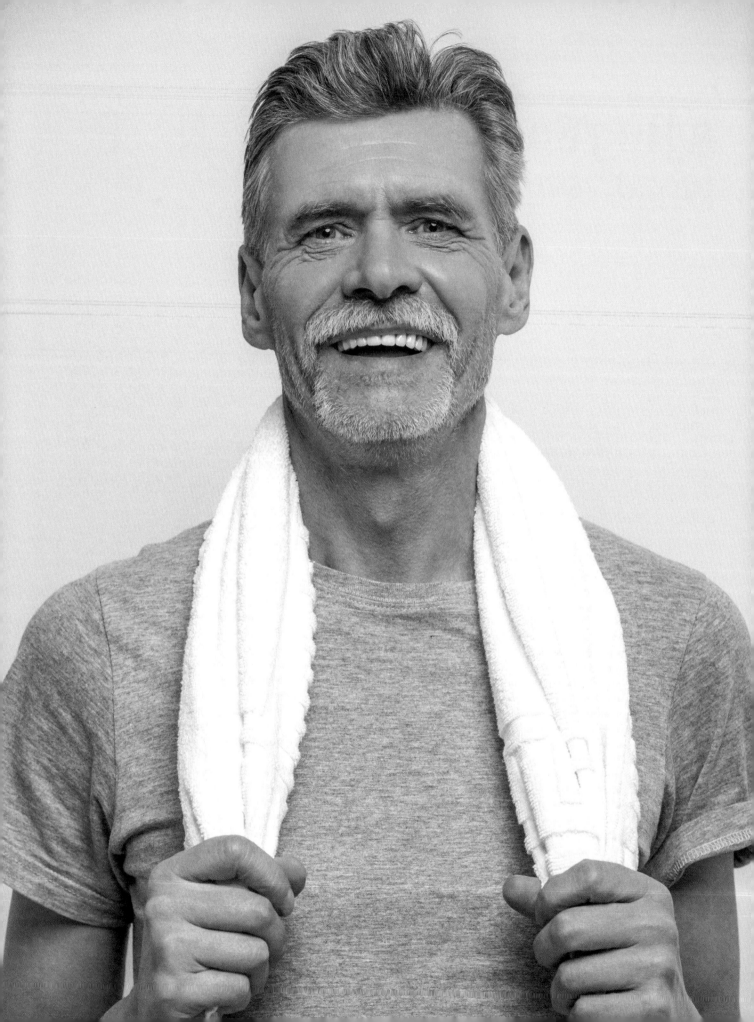

CHAPTER ONE

Aging Sooner, or Later
Which Will It Be?

GETTING OLDER isn't so bad, if you consider the alternative. But once you get past a certain age, what kind of shape you're in makes a huge difference to your enjoyment and quality of life—the two factors that, to my mind, get to the heart of what successful aging means.

Judging from my circle of friends and acquaintances, a lot of older people who stay fit, active, and healthy are enjoying more freedom and fun than they've had in years. No longer preoccupied with building a career and raising a family, many of them are busy going out with friends, traveling, and keeping up with hobbies or sports. To be sure, some have been temporarily sidelined by an illness, medical treatments, or nonelective surgery. But their generally good health and sensible lifestyles have usually helped them be resilient and get back to the way they were before.

For those who are steadily losing physical functionality, it's a different picture. If you know someone like this—perhaps a family member or a close friend— you know how heartbreaking it can be to watch someone's world shrinking as they grow weaker, stiffer, and slower, year by year. The less they do, the less they can do. It's a vicious cycle that only accelerates if nothing is done to reverse it. Daily activities like doing errands and fixing meals become more difficult. Aches and pains multiply, as do the risks of a serious illness or devastating fall.

When things reach the point where simple tasks become major stumbling blocks, living independently may no longer be an option. Too many people spend their "golden years" hobbled by immobility and pain—and in many cases it doesn't have to be that way.

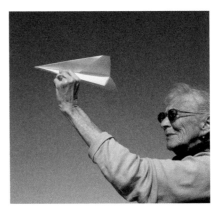

TO A SURPRISING DEGREE, HOW RAPIDLY YOU AGE IS UP TO YOU.

IN THIS CHAPTER

- *The aging process, deconstructed*

- *Why it's worth pushing back against old age*

- *The dangers of sitting*

- *How being active enriches your life*

BECAUSE WE'RE LIVING LONGER, MORE OF US WILL EXPERIENCE THE CHALLENGES OF EXTREME OLD AGE.

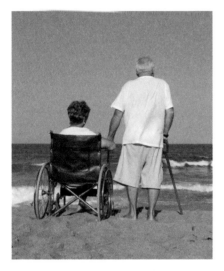

A SAD DOWNHILL SLIDE

A chance encounter brought all this home to me in a very personal way. Not long ago, while walking down an airport concourse to catch a flight home, I spotted someone resembling a former colleague I hadn't seen in some years. At first I thought I had to be mistaken. I knew that Bob was younger than I; by my reckoning, he was somewhere in his mid-sixties. But this man looked and moved like someone at least ten years older. He appeared frail and unsteady as he slowly shuffled onto the automated walkway, setting down his small carry on bag. You could see that every step was an effort, and he clutched the railing tightly for support.

As I waited at the end of the walkway, I saw that this was indeed my business associate from years past. "Well, look who's here," I said in greeting. "I haven't seen you in ages, Bob. How are things going?"

"Hi, Jim," he replied, looking a little startled as he stepped out of the flow of foot traffic. "Yes, you could say it's been a while. I'm okay, I guess."

"Just okay?" I asked, a little hesitant to pry.

"Well, I've had some setbacks lately. My knees are killing me, and I just can't seem to get around the way I used to. There's no way I would have made this trip if I didn't absolutely have to," Bob replied. He told me he was now completely retired and spent most of his time reading and watching TV. No longer able to navigate the stairs in the home he'd occupied for years, he'd recently moved in to a one-story house that he was having retrofitted with grab bars, a walk-in bathtub, and wider doorways to accommodate the wheelchair he might need down the road.

"Isn't there something else you can do?" I asked. "Have you tried physical therapy? Maybe some kind of exercise program?"

"Not really," he said. "You know me. I've never been the gym-rat type, and I certainly don't feel up to starting anything like that now."

I took a breath and forged ahead. "Forgive me for asking this...but would you be willing to give up an hour a day if it meant you could feel better and move more easily?" I asked, curious as to what his response would be.

"Of course I would!" he said without hesitation. "That's a no-brainer. I ache all over. Why would I choose to live like this if I could make things different?"

I didn't say what I was thinking: in a way, you did choose this, because making no effort to maintain or improve your fitness is also a choice, even if it's an unwitting one. If my old colleague had started investing just an hour a day in his mobility when he retired, his situation now might be quite different. Had he begun five or ten years earlier, the odds are he'd be in even better shape.

As if reading my mind, Bob said, with a heavy sigh, "It's too late now." Already inactive, housebound, and seemingly depressed, he evidently saw nothing ahead of him but a continued downward slide. With some expert advice and a program of regular activity, Bob could still turn things around. Regrettably, he couldn't even see how that was possible.

THE CASE FOR TAKING ACTION NOW

Let's face it: aging is unavoidable. Because we're living longer, more of us will experience the challenges of extreme old age. And there are no do-overs for years spent sitting at a desk or in front of a screen.

Like my old colleague, many older people seem to feel they are helpless in the face of their advancing years. They see physical change as something that happens to them—not as a process they have the power to harness or influence. To their way of thinking, creeping decrepitude is "normal" and to be expected once someone hits 65 or 70. This is a common mind-set, but one that's outdated and needs to change.

For one thing, the conventional definition of old age as beginning around age 65 is obsolete when many people that age might live another two decades or more. Medical researchers are moving toward a definition of old age based on measures of physical function—your fitness age—rather than just how many birthdays you've had.

The good news, as scientists are learning, is that we have a great deal more control over the aging process than many people think. You can't keep from aging, but you can do something about how rapidly you age. A growing body of research shows that being physically active can help you lower the risks of serious disease while sidestepping or postponing many of the most debilitating effects of old age. Some of the most compelling evidence of that comes from studies of older amateur athletes.

MANY OLDER PEOPLE SEE PHYSICAL CHANGE AS SOMETHING THAT HAPPENS TO THEM— NOT A PROCESS THEY HAVE THE POWER TO INFLUENCE.

THAT'S AN OUTDATED MIND-SET.

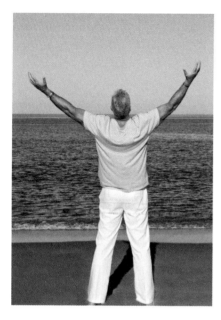

FITNESS ISN'T
A DESTINATION;
IT'S A WAY OF LIFE.

For example, one study of 5,000 older athletes in Norway found they typically had a fitness age that was 20 or more years younger than their chronological age. Another research effort in the U.S. evaluated 4,200 Senior Olympics participants who averaged 68 years of age. Remarkably, it found their average fitness age was 43—a 25-year difference! What's more, the effect was roughly the same for men as for women. People like these Olympians are living proof that someone who's 70 and fit may be physiologically younger than a 45-year-old who gets little or no exercise.

It's true that many older athletes have trained and competed for years, giving them a leg up on the rest of us. But research shows that exercise can also benefit aging adults who have been mostly sedentary. One of the biggest recent studies of that population followed 1,635 people who were between 70 and 89, had not been exercising, and were close to being infirm. After two and a half years, those who participated in a regular program of walking and light weight training were significantly less likely to have experienced episodes of physical disability or become permanently disabled.

Of course, there are no guarantees in life, and luck does play some role in all this. An illness or accident can strike at any time, no matter how fit someone may be. But that's all the more reason to make sure you're able to fully enjoy as many years of your life as you possibly can.

INVESTING IN YOUR FUTURE

If you're thinking about becoming more active, don't let the old bodybuilding, pumping-iron stereotypes put you off. A fitness program doesn't have to be grueling, complicated, or expensive. There are plenty of easy ways to get moving and even have fun in the process.

Experts generally agree that an effective program for adults of any age should include about 150 minutes of aerobic physical activity a week, as well as some muscle-strengthening activity at least twice a week. ("Aerobic" means physical activity that elevates your heart rate, makes you breathe harder than when you're at rest, and can be sustained for at least ten minutes.) Older adults who want to be functionally fit need activities that also address other dimensions of fitness, including flexibility and balance (see Chapter 4). My step-by-step program is designed to let you cover all those bases with a time commitment of one hour a day, six days a week.

When you think about it, the choice to invest in fitness, or not, isn't so different from the financial choices we make. We spend years saving and investing for retirement, choosing to forgo some purchases and pleasures for the sake of greater security later on. If you now decide to invest just an hour a day in your physical functioning, you'll be choosing to make your later years the very best they can be.

So ask yourself these questions:

- *What do you want your life to be like when you are 70 or 80?*

- *Are you willing to spend an hour a day now to raise the odds of having the future you want?*

If so, this is the book for you!

A ONE-HOUR WORKOUT TAKES UP ONLY 4% OF YOUR DAY.

*As you get older,
the questions come down
to about two or three.
How long? And what do
I do with the time
I've got left?*

DAVID BOWIE

The Trouble With Being Sedentary

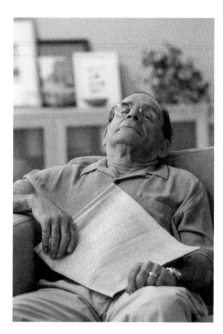

Let's not turn a blind eye to the hazards of being a couch potato. As detailed below, the sedentary life is killing us, and robbing our older years of vitality and enjoyment in the process. According to 2015 surveys by the Centers for Disease Control and Prevention (CDC), only about half of all U.S. adults get the level of aerobic activity experts recommend. Less than 22 percent meet the guidelines for both aerobic and muscle-strengthening activity, and those figures drop to just 15 percent of those in the 65-to-74 age bracket and less than 10 percent of those over 75. It doesn't help that more than a third of U.S. adults qualify as obese (not just overweight), making them even less likely to be active. Here are some of the more dire consequences of being inactive:

Higher risks of serious disease. Researchers have tied the sedentary life to a litany of serious health threats, including leading killers like heart disease, cancer, chronic respiratory disease, diabetes, and stroke. Recent studies have concluded that too much sitting leads to 92,000 cases of cancer in the U.S. annually, and a 40 percent increase in the odds of dying from any cause in a given year. And on a global level, a 2011 Harvard Medical School study found a lack of activity was responsible for one in ten deaths worldwide, or more than five million a year, outstripping mortality from smoking. Of the $3 trillion or so the U.S. spends on health care each year, an astonishing 86 percent is directed toward ongoing medical conditions that are partly or mostly the result of lifestyle choices.

Less mobility and physical function. "Use it or lose it" isn't just a catch-phrase. Older people who don't work on their strength and agility find it progressively harder to get through their daily routines. They have more aches and pains, take smaller steps, and move more slowly and cautiously. Basic movements like navigating stairs or getting in and out of chairs are harder and take longer. Chores like cleaning and grocery shopping become exhausting. One study of people over 74 years of age found that 28 percent of males and 76 percent of females couldn't lift even ten pounds, less than the weight of a bag of groceries. The more difficult daily living becomes for older people, the less they're likely to do, making things even worse.

More falls and injuries. On average, one out of three Americans over 65 sustains a fall each year, many of them serious. Falls annually lead to an estimated 250,000 hip fractures and are the sixth leading cause of death among people over 65. Many people don't realize that balance begins to decline not in middle age, but when we're in our twenties. With age, we lose function in our *proprio-ceptors*, the sensory nerve endings that enable us to sense where our body is in space, and in the parts of the inner ear that relay information about gravity and motion. Add to that age-related losses in vision, muscle strength, and flexibility, and you can see why falling is one of the biggest hazards older people face.

Loss of independence. According to research by AARP (the American Association of Retired Persons), nine out of ten seniors want to stay in their own homes through retirement, and only 14 percent expect to need day-to-day assistance or ongoing health care at any point. The reality check: A recent study of 8,000 older American found that nearly 40 percent of them needed help to get around or accomplish the basic tasks of daily living. Another 25 percent could only do these things with the help of devices like canes or bathroom grab bars. Older people who are in denial about their future prospects are less likely to take steps that will help them preserve their mobility and independence.

No quote I've ever seen sums it all up better than the one from Edward Stanley, a 19th-century British statesman. As he said in a speech more than 140 years ago, "Those who think they have not time for bodily exercise will sooner or later have to find time for illness."

FATAL ATTRACTION?

THE PLEASURES OF TV ARE ADDICTIVE.

But spending hours a day in front of the tube can be downright dangerous. One study found that people who watch seven or more hours a day had a **61% greater risk of dying prematurely** than those who watched an hour or less.

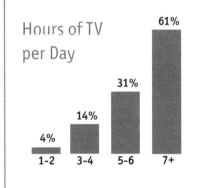

Hours of TV per Day

- 1-2: 4%
- 3-4: 14%
- 5-6: 31%
- 7+: 61%

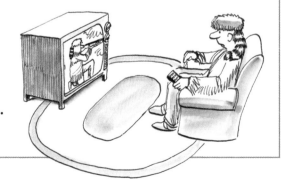

YOUR FAVORITE CHAIR IS NOT YOUR FRIEND

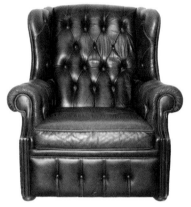

THOUSANDS OF YEARS AGO, our ancestors were nomadic hunter-gatherers, constantly on the move in search of food, shelter, and safety from predators. Odds are that your grandparents got plenty of physical activity, too. Before 1920 or so, most Americans still worked hard on farms or ranches, and less than half of all U.S. families owned an automobile. The idea of having to allot time to "exercise" would have seemed very strange to people who sat down mainly to eat.

Today we spend most of our waking hours sitting, whether at a desk, in a car, or in front of the TV. Many of us don't even turn the pages in books anymore, and it's been decades since we got up from the couch to change the TV channel.

A rising tide of evidence points to excessive sitting as a scourge of our culture—one that kills more people than smoking. It has been linked to obesity, diabetes, heart disease, liver disease, and cancer. In fact, researchers have estimated that too much sitting leads to 92,000 cases

of cancer in the U.S. annually. One of the largest recent studies found that people who sit in a chair for 11 hours or more a day increased their risks of premature death, from any cause, by more than 40 percent. What's more, the impact of sitting was so pronounced that even a vigorous exercise session the same day wasn't enough to offset it.

Long periods of sitting are also terrible for your mobility. Besides leaving you with progressively tighter hips, habitual sitting causes poor posture, back problems, and degeneration of muscles. That said, getting a standing desk isn't necessarily a panacea, either. When it comes to avoiding heart problems and diabetes, the issue isn't so much whether you're sitting or standing upright,

scientists say. The real problem is immobility. When your muscles are working, their contractions trigger biochemical reactions that help keep your blood sugar, insulin, and cholesterol profiles in check. If your muscles aren't contracting, your metabolism isn't working as it should—and if that happens for hours every day, the health risks quickly mount.

The best way to reduce the risks of immobility, experts say, is to take frequent breaks and move around. That will help keep your metabolism humming along on an even keel. Studies show that even fidgeting helps! So when you're at a desk or in a chair, get up for five minutes every half hour or so. If you're standing, take time out to stretch and move around. Programming reminders into your smartphone or laptop is one way to make sure you don't get absorbed in something and let hours go by without moving.

The best preventive medicine we have can be summed up in two words: *JUST MOVE!*

THE DOWNWARD SPIRAL OF AGING

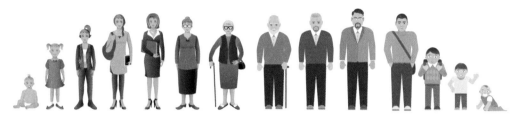

Aging doesn't happen overnight. It's a gradual process that starts long before the first gray hairs and accelerates with the years if you don't counteract it with exercise.

20s BALANCE starts to degrade, as the body's spatial sensory receptors gradually become less effective.

30s AEROBIC CAPACITY (maximal oxygen consumption), a key measure of cardiovascular function, begins to drop by 5 to 15 percent per decade; this makes the heart beat faster and work less efficiently.

BONE DENSITY DECREASES 1 percent per year after age 35, more rapidly for women after menopause, leaving bones weaker and more brittle. Women may lose 25 to 30 percent of bone mass by age 60.

40s MEMORY AND REASONING POWER begin a slow decline.

50s LOSS OF MUSCLE MASS accelerates. About 10 percent is already gone; expect to lose another 15 percent per decade.

60s WEIGHT GAIN, averaging ten pounds per decade from the age of 25, has mounting effects. With less muscle tissue, metabolic rate is reduced and fewer calories are burned.

BODY FAT increases as a share of total body mass, rising from an average of 25 to 43 percent for women and 18 to 38 percent for men in their sixties and seventies, and more fat is deposited around vital organs. Being in the upper range triples the risk of heart disease and stroke.

70s BALANCE PROBLEMS and falls increase. One-third of adults over 65 will fall at least once every year.

MUSCULAR STRENGTH drops with muscle mass after age 50; adults over 70 may have only 50 percent of the strength of young adults.

80s FLEXIBILITY of the lower back and hips has declined by three to four inches, based on "sit and reach" tests, restricting movements.

MAXIMAL OXYGEN INTAKE eventually drops below levels required for independent movement.

DEPENDENCE ON OTHERS is common after age 80, typically involving several years of partial disability and up to a year of full dependency.

The Good News

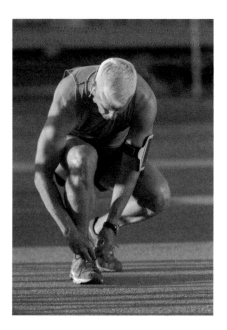

EXERCISE IS THE ONE ANTIAGING TREATMENT THAT IS ENTIRELY IN YOUR POWER.

On one thing the experts agree: ***exercise is the most effective way to slow down the aging process.*** Moreover, it's the one preventive step that can be low in cost and is entirely in your power. Being physically active helps prevent disease by increasing blood flow, improving cardiovascular function, and helping to normalize the body's blood sugar and insulin levels. Exercise has been shown to reduce chronic systemic inflammation, a common autoimmune reaction that is a risk factor for some cancers and can cause a wide array of other health problems, including rheumatoid arthritis and heart disease. Weight-bearing exercise can also help strengthen bones that otherwise become less dense and more brittle with age.

This is not to say that exercise is a magic bullet banishing all physical ailments. It cannot restore tissue that has been destroyed. But it's true that those who exercise live longer than others, and they typically live much better lives. Exercise has been shown to help older people enjoy good health, functional capacity, and quality of life for a much longer period than those who don't keep moving. As the saying goes, "It's not the years in your life that count. It's the life in your years."

Beyond helping to reduce or prevent some of the most disabling effects of aging, staying active is a way to:

Look and feel younger. When you think about it, nothing telegraphs "old" as clearly as stooped posture, a shuffling gait, and slow, listless movements. A good workout gets your blood pumping, leaving you with a burst of energy and a healthy glow. It's like an instant antiaging treatment. Over time, a good exercise program will help you stand taller and move with more confidence and energy. Plenty of celebrities have gray hair and wrinkled skin—think of Sean Connery, Judi Dench, Richard Gere, Helen Mirren, or Harrison Ford. But they still project a youthful vigor and sparkle that's ageless.

Help control your weight. The formula for weight loss is simple: ***you've got to burn more calories than you take in.*** Physical activity can certainly help you boost your calorie expenditure. But let's be clear: exercise is just one element of a weight-loss program. Controlling caloric intake is also critical, because it might take an hour or more of vigorous activity to burn off that jelly donut you couldn't resist. When it comes to ***maintaining*** a healthy weight, however, regular exercise is vital. According to the CDC, "evidence shows the only way to maintain weight loss is to be engaged in regular physical activity." Activities that build muscle, like strength training, will also increase your metabolic rate so you burn more calories even when you're at rest.

KNOW YOUR FITNESS AGE

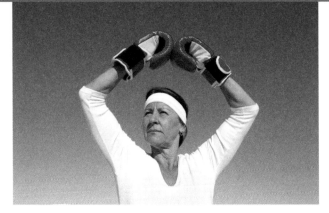

AGE IS ONLY A NUMBER, the saying goes. And it's certainly true that your level of fitness isn't determined by how many birthdays you've had. But there is another number that does matter.

Scientists can now measure your fitness age, which has proved to be a better predictor of life span than your chronological age. What's more, with regular exercise you can actually turn back the clock and lower your fitness age.

As large-scale studies of senior athletes have shown, people who are active may have the physical function of a much younger person. Take, for example, the 4,200 senior athletes who competed at the 2015 Senior Olympics. Although their chronological age averaged 68, their average fitness age was just 43—a full quarter century younger!

Methods of calculating fitness age were developed by researchers at the Norwegian University of Science and Technology based on large-scale studies of people between the ages of 20 and 90. One of the key determinants of fitness age is VO_2 *max*, which measures aerobic capacity, your body's ability to take in and utilize oxygen. The researchers also factored in a variety of health parameters relating to risks of serious disease, including waist circumference, resting heart rate, and exercise habits.

To precisely measure your VO_2 max, you will need to be tested on a high-tech treadmill at a sports medicine lab. There they'll ask you to work up to your maximum exertion level while wearing a device that measures your oxygen consumption and carbon dioxide output. That's not convenient for most people, and pushing exertion levels to the max may be unsafe for those with a heart condition or other chronic health problems.

You can easily estimate your fitness age by going online. At *worldfitnesslevel.org*, you'll find the questionnaire developed by the Norwegian University of Science and Technology team. It uses an algorithm to roughly calculate your fitness age by comparing your answers with data collected from 55,000 research subjects. Another useful resource is *shapesense.com,* which offers four different ways to estimate your VO_2 max. Its set of fitness and exercise calculators also includes ways to estimate heart rate, basal metabolic rate, caloric burn, and more.

Finding out your fitness age is a great way to kick off a new fitness program, giving yourself an added shot of motivation, encouragement, or both. Who says you can't turn back the clock?

Give your brain a boost. It has long been known that exercise increases blood flow, which means your brain will almost immediately function better after a workout. But researchers have found another mechanism behind the heightened mental focus and clarity we often feel after exercising. Physical activity stimulates the release of a protein called *brain-derived neurotrophic factor,* or BDNF, which encourages the growth of nerve cells, strengthens neural connections, and protects them from damage. This may help explain why older people who get regular, moderate exercise like walking are less likely to suffer from dementia, Alzheimer's, or Parkinson's disease. Recent studies also suggest that a combination of strength and aerobic training can help improve cognitive functioning by reversing some age-related shrinkage of the hippocampus, the part of the brain associated with memory and learning.

Avoid falls and injuries. Falls are epidemic among the older population, and they can trigger a cascade of serious and even life-threatening consequences. Yet for some reason even professional trainers often overlook the importance of training the body's balance mechanisms, which gradually lose effectiveness from early adulthood on. To keep from falling, you also need core strength (think lower back and abdominals), lower-body strength, and flexibility. Simple strength and balance exercises, many of which can be done at home, can go a long way toward helping older people stay solidly on their feet. Fitness training can also help you get in the habit of moving more mindfully and cautiously—the first line of defense against falling.

Ease chronic pain. Physical activity may be the last thing on the minds of people suffering from chronic pain due to back or joint problems, cancer, or autoimmune diseases like rheumatoid arthritis, multiple sclerosis, and fibromyalgia. But it turns out that too much rest can worsen pain over time, as inactivity leads to even weaker, tighter muscles, more stiffness in joints, and more focus on pain. Conversely, simply moving the body can be good therapy for pain.

Studies have shown that people who get regular exercise manage their pain much better than those who are inactive. For one thing, physical activity stimulates the body to produce natural morphine-like painkillers. Movement therapies like gentle stretching, water aerobics, yoga, and tai chi also help those in pain to relax, reducing the release of stress hormones that cause systemic inflammation and worsen pain. It's important to remember, though, that no one kind of exercise is right for everyone seeking pain relief. If that's your situation, be sure to consult a doctor or physical therapist before embarking on any exercise program.

Prevent osteoporosis. An estimated 12 million people over 50 have brittle, porous bones, increasing their risk of fracture. Another 47 million people have low bone mass, known as *osteopenia*, and are at risk for developing osteoporosis. And this is not just a concern for women; one in four men over age 50 can expect to have a fracture due to osteoporosis at some point in life. Because bone is living tissue, weight-bearing exercise can help stimulate bone growth. While swimming and bicycling are good for your health, your bones need to feel the effects of gravity if they're to grow thicker, denser, and stronger. Thus, activities like walking and strength training can help reduce osteoporosis risks. Your doctor may recommend calcium and vitamin D supplements, too.

Counter anxiety and depression. Exercise is a proven mood-lifter, and the more scientists learn about it, the more they understand why. Physical activity stimulates neurotransmitters such as endorphins (the brain's "feel-good" chemical), serotonin, dopamine, glutamate, and gamma-aminobutyric acid (GABA). So while people who are depressed often ask for medication first, many clinicians counsel them to try exercise instead of or alongside an antidepressant drug. One fascinating study published in the journal *Psychosomatic Medicine* found that depressed people treated with exercise alone were far more likely to be depression-free six months after the end of the trial than those treated with medication. What's more, the benefits of physical activity come with no side effects and begin almost right away! Researchers say that mood typically begins to brighten about ten minutes into an exercise session.

Enjoy a better sex life. If it's motivation you want, think about this: physical activity produces chemical substances that make a woman's body more sensitive to touch and stimulate sex hormones in both men and women. Exercise also gets your cardiovascular system moving, sending more blood flow to all the right places. And while I wouldn't claim that exercise makes Viagra obsolete, studies show that the more physically active men are, the higher their reported quality of sexual function. Strength training has been shown to increase levels of growth hormone and testosterone, the hormone of male arousal. Overall, being fit will give you more stamina, boost your energy, and help you feel better about your body—all important ingredients for a healthy libido.

Reduce your need for prescription drugs. Americans use more prescription drugs than people in any other developed country—nearly $1,000 worth per capita each year. A 2013 study by the Mayo Clinic found that nearly 70 percent of the U.S. population is on at least one prescription drug, half take at least two, and 20 percent take five or more. Experts say that getting more exercise could

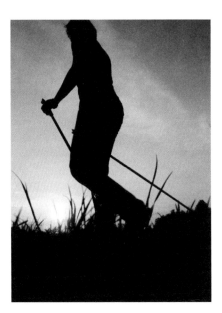

SIMPLY MOVING THE BODY CAN BE GOOD THERAPY FOR PAIN.

ONE OF LIFE'S
GREATEST MOMENTS
IS REALIZING THAT
TWO WEEKS AGO,
YOUR BODY COULDN'T
DO WHAT IT JUST DID.

help many people take fewer pharmaceuticals, saving money and suffering fewer side effects in the bargain. The natural painkillers produced by physical activity could help people cut back on their use of antidepressants and opioid painkillers, which are the second and third most commonly prescribed types of drugs in the U.S. (antibiotics are first). Exercise also lowers cholesterol and improves cardiovascular health. According to the Mayo Clinic, becoming more active may also lower systolic blood pressure about as much as some blood pressure medications.

Gain confidence and pride in yourself. I had no idea how big a difference getting fit would make to my self-image and general outlook on life. Feeling and looking better is an obvious boon. Who doesn't like to hear people exclaim, "You look amazing!"? I also like being able to say, "No, thanks" when the hotel bellman offers to carry my suitcase. It's good to know I'm plenty strong enough to take care of the routine physical tasks that come my way. Now I walk through my day straight and tall, with my head held high.

Best of all is the sense of accomplishment I feel. I set some ambitious fitness goals for myself. Through persistence, determination, and a little help from my friends, I've met them all. Now I know I've got what it takes to make big changes in my life. Becoming fit has given me a feeling of personal power and a renewed sense of possibility. If I can do this, what else can I do?

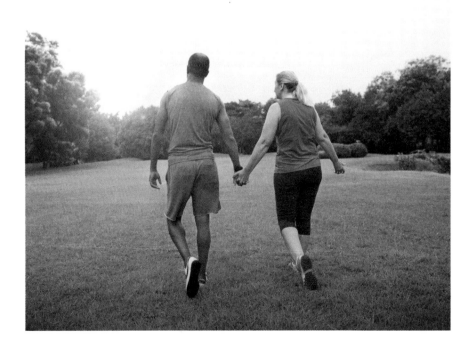

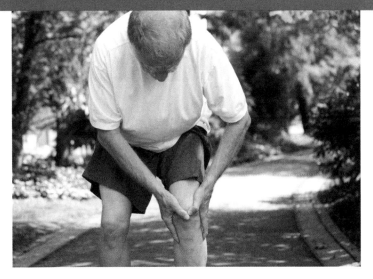

IF YOU SUFFER from some form of arthritis—as about half of all Americans 65 or older do—sitting still may feel like the best policy. Being plagued by aching knees, hips, shoulders, ankles, elbows, or wrists can blunt anyone's appetite for exercise. Why get off the couch when every move hurts?

Unfortunately, researchers tell us, controlling your arthritis pain by limiting activity only makes things worse. Large-scale studies have shown that when arthritis sufferers are inactive, the disease eventually takes over. The less that people with arthritis move, the more function they lose. Their pain tends to intensify, partly because leg muscles weaken, putting even more strain on joints.

Inactivity often leads to chronic health problems like heart disease or type 2 diabetes. And when people are forced to give up activities they enjoy, or can't handle the tasks of daily living, depression often follows, making them even less likely to move. It's a vicious cycle that explains why arthritis is the most common cause of disability in the U.S.

Moderate exercise, on the other hand, can make a big difference by helping to keep joints lubricated and mobile, increasing function and reducing pain. When the American College of Rheumatology studied the nonprofit Arthritis Foundation's six-week Walk With Ease program, they found that regular walking decreased disability and arthritis symptoms.

If arthritis is keeping you from being active in the ways you'd like to be, find some lower-impact activities you can do, like walking, swimming, water aerobics, or bicycling. Tai chi, with its gentle, fluid movements, is an ancient form of exercise often recommended for those with arthritis. Try some options and find what works for you. You may also be a candidate for joint replacement surgery, which is becoming commonplace. More than 757,000 total knee replacements and 512,000 total hip replacements were performed in the U.S. in 2011. According to the American Academy of Orthopaedic Surgeons, 90 percent of those who have the surgery report significantly less pain following rehab and are often able to resume activities like golf and walking.

If you don't have arthritis, consider yourself lucky. You can lower your risks of developing the disease by keeping off or losing excess weight, being careful not to injure your joints, and strengthening muscles to give your joints more support.

ARE WE JUST PLAIN *LAZY?*

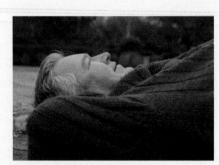

Too little exercise. Too many inches around the middle. And all the aches and pains that go along with being stiffer, weaker, and flabbier than we want to be. So many of us struggle with the same garden-variety physical issues as we age.

Evolutionary biologists tell us that's really no surprise. The human body evolved over several million years to deal with a set of conditions completely different from modern lifestyles. In essence, we're operating with Stone Age bodies in a high-tech world.

That certainly sheds light on our food addictions. Babies are born with a strong liking for sweet flavors and an aversion to bitter ones, an evolutionary advantage that helped humans avoid toxic berries and rotten meat. The body's need for a certain amount of sodium, which helps control the balance of internal fluids, could be behind our love of salty munchables like pretzels and tortilla chips. The average American today gets a whopping 50 percent more sodium than the recommended daily intake, health surveys show. More than three-quarters of that is from processed foods, including some that don't taste salty, like bread, cookies, and condiments. But since sodium would have been much scarcer in the hunter-gatherer diets of our Paleo forebears, our tastes may still be geared to helping us avoid salt deficiencies.

Our cravings for foods high in fats and carbohydrates are also inborn, a legacy of the time when our ancestors needed all the calories they could get. Today most people in developed nations have the opposite problem: how to "just say no" to French fries and ice cream. That's tough to do when food is always at hand and we're constantly bombarded with cues encouraging us to eat. And don't think the food industry hasn't capitalized on our natural taste preferences in every way possible!

As for being couch potatoes, scientists say our brains are hardwired for that, too. Although our bodies are designed to be working machines, Paleolithic people couldn't afford to expend energy needlessly. Once their basic survival requirements were met, they needed to be as lazy as possible.

In a world where our fingers can do most of the walking, that's a difficult tendency to overcome. One study found that when people were given a choice between an escalator or stairs, only 3 percent opted for the stairs, even if they were no farther away. If Aboriginal Australians or Kalahari Bushmen had escalators, they would probably use them, too.

Then there's the problem of expanding waistlines. Here, too, our natural bias toward inactivity (call it "energy conservation") works against us as we age. Did you know that Americans gain an average of one pound a year after the age of 25? That adds up to 35 pounds of excess weight by the age of 60!

We're losing the battle of the bulge, and it's not only because of what we eat, or how much. It's also because our metabolisms grow more sluggish as we steadily lose muscle with age. Unless we are actively building lean muscle mass through physical work or exercise, it declines at the rate of 2 to 4 percent every year after the age of 25 or so. Since muscle burns more calories than other kinds of tissue, less muscle translates into less calorie expenditure for any kind of activity. Think about what that means: if you're not exercising to build muscle and rev up your metabolism, you can stick to the same diet that kept you slim and lean in your twenties and still watch your weight creep up year by year.

We can take some comfort in the idea that our inherited instincts help explain our behavior patterns. But that doesn't mean they excuse them. *Homo sapiens* has also evolved with big brains we can use to recognize and counteract our natural leanings toward an inactive, overfed way of life. The more you know, the more you understand why it makes sense to focus on fitness.

THE ONLY EXERCISE SOME PEOPLE GET IS JUMPING TO CONCLUSIONS, RUNNING UP BILLS, STRETCHING THE TRUTH, BENDING OVER BACKWARD, LYING DOWN ON THE JOB, SIDESTEPPING RESPONSIBILITY, AND PUSHING THEIR LUCK.

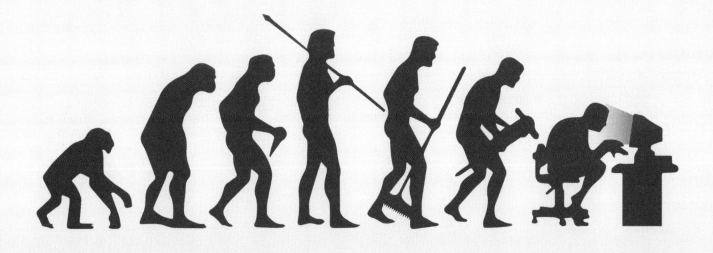

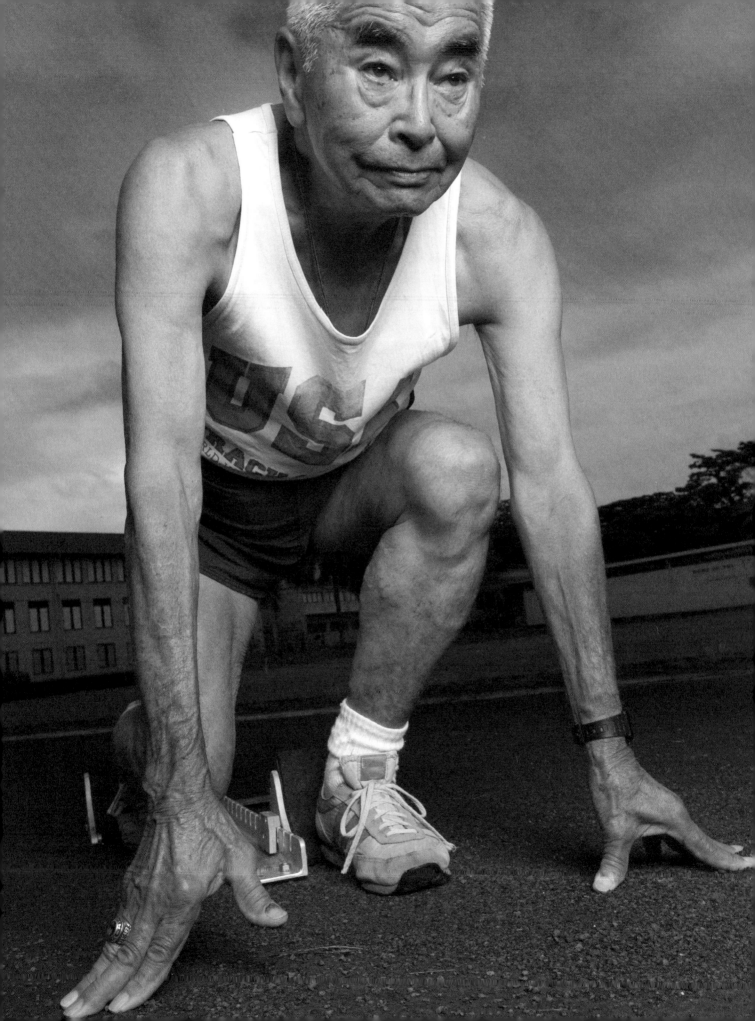

CHAPTER TWO

How to Succeed at Fitness
Mind-set Makes the Difference

IF YOU'RE LIKE MOST PEOPLE, you've more than once resolved to exercise and get fit. And, if you're like most of us, those resolutions have usually gone by the wayside. Research suggests that about 75 percent of people who make New Year's resolutions will stick with them no longer than a week. Only about 40 percent stay the course for as long as six months.

When you're 30-something, it's easy to give yourself a pass about a failure to follow through; at that age you're probably not being nagged by aches and pains, and you can always tell yourself there's still plenty of time to get on the fitness track. But when you're in your fifties, sixties, or seventies, the ticking of the clock is more insistent. The aging process is like a freight train that's rolling downhill. If you want to apply the brakes, you can't afford to delay. Your best chance is taking action *now.*

Believe me, I've been one of those who vowed to get fit and soon slid back into my old habits. But things are different now. I have finally made fitness a way of life—and I promise you that as long as I'm still upright, that's not going to change. It's all about getting motivated, and staying motivated day in and day out, even when you're too busy or "don't feel like it." Occasional bouts of exercise won't improve your physical functioning, and may put you at risk for an injury. *Consistency is the key.*

In short, if you want to be fit and strong for life, you've got to invest an hour of honest effort toward that goal, six days a week—and I won't pretend that's easy. Kelly McGonigal, a Ph.D. health psychologist at Stanford University, explains why fitness and health resolutions can be especially tough to stick with. As she told the TED blog, "Everything we think of as requiring willpower is usually a competition between two conflicting selves. There's a part of you who is looking to the long-term and thinking about certain goals, and then another part of you that has a completely different agenda and wants to maximize current pleasure and minimize current stress, pain and discomfort."

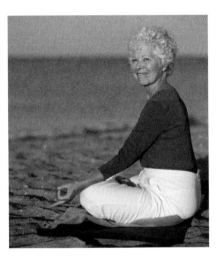

YOU CAN'T HELP GETTING OLDER, BUT YOU DON'T HAVE TO GET OLD.

IN THIS CHAPTER

- *Why the "small steps" approach makes sense*

- *How to forge the habits you want*

- *Finding your inner athlete*

- *The ultimate motivator*

THE AGING PROCESS IS LIKE A FREIGHT TRAIN THAT'S ROLLING DOWNHILL. IF YOU WANT TO APPLY THE BRAKES, YOU NEED TO DO IT *NOW.*

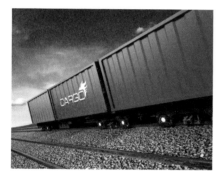

Luckily, there's a way to completely bypass the inner tug-of-war between long-term health and short-term ease. The conflict disappears when working out is something you **want** to do—a part of your life that's genuinely enjoyable. If you've ever experienced the burst of vitality that follows a good workout, you'll know what I'm talking about. Once you start exercising regularly, and notice how much younger, stronger, and just plain good you feel, you'll never want to go back to the old you. What's more, you'll know that you can set out to change your life, and actually accomplish it over the long haul!

For most people, the most challenging parts are getting started and moving past the initial hump. That's why I've designed a step-by-step program that helps you ease into the fitness habit, slowly but surely. I've also pulled together the six secrets that helped me succeed at fitness. I promise they can help you, too.

MAKE A PLEDGE TO YOURSELF

If you really, truly want to slow down the aging process, you need to build fitness into your life. Ideally, it should become as much a part of your daily routine as brushing your teeth. To help bolster your commitment and resolve:

Put it in writing. For my own pledge I wrote, "I want to eliminate my aches and pains and become as fit as I can possibly be—and I'm willing to do whatever it takes to get there." You might gear your own pledge to what would most motivate you. (See the end of this chapter for some food for thought.)

Commit to a specific action plan. It should spell out exactly what you intend to do and on what time line. For example, you might say, "I am going to work out with a personal trainer three times a week." Allowing for two weeks of vacation, that adds up to 150 workouts a year. Follow through on that plan and you can't help but grow more fit.

Make it a priority. Think of your exercise sessions as "me time"—one of the most important things you do for yourself. Put them on the calendar in ink, and don't let anything intervene that isn't an equally high priority. If you must skip a walk or workout and can't reschedule, don't fret about it. Just hit the "resume" button and keep going.

Use positive peer pressure. Tell your partner and your friends what you're doing, and ask them to give you encouragement and reminders of your intentions. Better yet, enlist a buddy or neighbor to walk or work out with you. The people around you can help expand your reservoir of motivation.

SET REALISTIC GOALS

Enthusiasm is great, but a program that's too intense or ambitious at the outset is likely to fizzle, cause injuries, or both. Remember, fitness is an ongoing process. There's no finish line; all that matters is that you keep advancing over time. You'll be more successful if you start from where you are and concentrate on making small, incremental improvements. The program in this book is designed to help you do just that.

My advice is to:

Concentrate on functional fitness. To keep old age at bay, focus on practical fitness objectives—that is, maintaining your mobility and being physically able to accomplish the things you need and want to do in your daily life. Don't let ego or vanity be the drivers. As you become more fit, you'll feel better, reduce stress, and gain confidence—and that's an unbeatable recipe for looking great, too.

Compete only with yourself. Why discourage yourself or risk injury by trying to match someone else? Other people may be at different stages of training, work out with different goals, or have different strengths and weaknesses than you. Concentrating on your own goals and progress is the surest way to forge ahead.

Make the most of the body you have. Not everyone is born with a naturally lean, athletic physique. But just about anyone can become more fit, regardless of body type. If your fitness goals include losing weight and firming up, that's great, just so long as dissatisfaction with your body doesn't stand in your way. Accepting who you are and where you are in life will help you reach your fitness potential.

Stick with the basics. Forget about the fads, and avoid information overload—there's just too much confusing and conflicting advice out there. While science keeps learning more about fitness, the fundamental principles really haven't changed all that much. Keeping it simple will help you stay focused.

Expect obstacles and reversals. Things happen. You might be temporarily sidelined by a cold, or distracted by a family situation. But don't let lapses derail you. Just get back to your program and keep going. You'll make up for lost time faster than you might think.

IDEALLY, FITNESS BECOMES AS MUCH A PART OF YOUR DAILY ROUTINE AS BRUSHING YOUR TEETH.

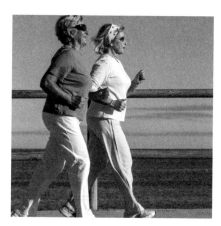

MOTIVATION GETS
YOU STARTED.
HABIT KEEPS YOU
COMING BACK.

GET IN THE HABIT

Build in reminders, routines, and rewards. There's a science to forming new habits, and researchers have found that three "Rs" are key.

- First, you need a *reminder.* That can be an entry on your calendar or some physical cue, like laying out your workout clothes the night before. You might post your written pledge, your list of exercises, or an inspiring photograph on the refrigerator, where you'll see it as you make your morning coffee. Having an appointment to walk with a friend or work out with a trainer is ideal.

- Then there is the *routine*—the behavior you want to incorporate consistently. You'll be more successful if you start building your new habit around something that's not too difficult. That's why the program in this book starts with stretching and walking. Making physical activity part of your daily routine is the most important first step. Another simple but highly effective tactic is to link the new behavior you want with a habit that's already firmly established. For example, you could decide to do your stretching routine right after your morning shower, or before you check your email. The good news is that success breeds more success. As you repeat your walk or your workout, your brain builds a network of neural connections around the behavior—and the more you repeat it, the stronger those connections will become.

- Ah, the *reward!* A good workout usually leaves an afterglow of energy and well-being. You will also have the satisfaction of giving yourself a big thumbs-up: "I did it!" This is a great time to reinforce your self-image as a person of strength and determination. If you want an added shot of motivation, give yourself a post-workout payoff, like a new magazine or a piece of dark chocolate. And there's nothing wrong with "bribing" yourself with a movie or a new pair of shoes if you do your targeted number of workouts for the month. Whatever gets results!

Join a gym. It's certainly possible to work out at home if you're motivated and knowledgeable. But a gym provides a structure and setting you'll get nowhere else. It's the place where you put everything else aside and concentrate on how you are moving. A well-equipped gym will give you a variety of workout options, so you keep challenging your body and don't get bored. It will also put you in the midst of a community of people who are pursuing the same goals as you.

Adjust your mental habits. If you groan inwardly at the prospect of getting off the couch and hitting the walking trail or the gym, work on your mind-set first. Instead of giving in to automatic reactions like "I hate exercise" or "I'm too out of shape for this," cultivate a positive, can-do attitude.

- Remind yourself how much better you'll feel right after your session. Some rewards are immediate!

- Use the power of visualization. Imagine oxygen pumping, blood flowing, and energy coursing through your body as you move. Think of all the other things you'll have the energy to do. Picture yourself as a fitness warrior ("My name is Spartacus!") or an Amazon—strong, disciplined, confident.

- Think in terms of moving up a spiral. Don't look to the metaphorical mountaintop; concentrate instead on taking the next step or doing the next movement. Do that one thing, and you can probably do another.

- Smile! Scientists have discovered that you'll enjoy exercising more if you act like you're having fun while doing it. While we all know that emotions can affect our facial expressions, research shows that it also works the other way, too.

Have a fallback position. We all have those days when we have low energy or just don't feel like working out. Instead of breaking the habit by skipping your regular walk or workout, scale it back. Walk half the distance, do exercises that are easier, or spend more time stretching rather than doing strength training. Doing something is always better than doing nothing.

DO SOMETHING
TODAY THAT YOUR
FUTURE SELF WILL
THANK YOU FOR.

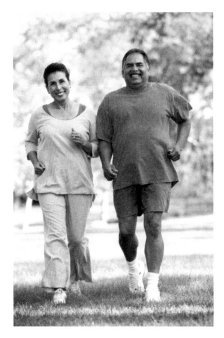

GIVE IT YOUR BEST EFFORT

Exercise is like most things in life: you get out of it what you put into it. Think of yourself as the kind of person who is mentally strong and determined to give your best. Then strive to be that person in your workouts. I promise you will come away with a genuine sense of pride, and others will recognize and respect you as someone who gives it your all.

Be focused and present. If you are tuned in to your body and the movement, you will be more engaged. You will also be able to pay more attention to exercise form, which is all-important if you want to avoid injury and get the full benefits of what you're doing (see Chapter 7). You may see others chatting on cell phones or burning up workout time with small talk. Don't let that be you—not if you're serious about getting results.

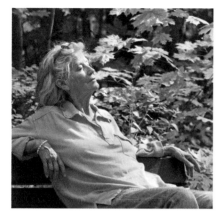

BE ACCOUNTABLE
TO YOURSELF.
YESTERDAY, YOU
SAID "TOMORROW."

Go for quality, not quantity. We tend to think in terms of the outcome of a movement—lifting that dumbbell, touching your toes, logging 20 minutes on a cardio machine. Yet the effectiveness of physical training depends less on accomplishing these tasks than on the quality and intensity of the effort we put into it. What matters isn't the output but the input. If you're exercising with poor posture or "cheating" by calling on muscles that shouldn't really play a role in the movement, you're not accomplishing what you set out to do.

Spend a little time doing what's hard. While we all have physical weaknesses and imbalances, it's human nature to focus on our strengths. We often gravitate to the exercises we can do more easily while skipping ones we find harder. But if you really want to improve, you must be willing to step out of your comfort zone. Make sure your workout includes at least one or two exercises that challenge you and target your areas of weakness.

KEEP PROGRESSING

Some people like to get in an exercise routine and stay there, never varying what they do or even the order they do it in. But that flies in the face of how exercise works. In essence, exercise challenges the musculoskeletal, cardiovascular, and respiratory systems of your body. When a particular challenge is repeated over and over, your body makes positive adaptations, increasing the capacity and efficiency of its systems. If you keep it up, your body adjusts and the exercise gets easier—but your physical gains also reach a plateau. Varying your routines, adding repetitions, or gradually increasing weight as your strength grows will all stimulate positive new adaptations that increase your overall fitness.

Ongoing improvements in fitness are especially important to older adults who want to keep the functionality they have while regaining the strength, conditioning, flexibility, and balance they may have lost. Who knows? You might even find yourself in better shape at 70 or 75 than you were at 45 or 50. That was certainly true for me.

Aim for slow, steady progress. By no means am I suggesting that you should try to make advances in every exercise or every dimension of fitness at once. Don't overdo it! Trying to do too much, too fast, can only lead to strain or injury. You'll get better results in the long run if you make small improvements in one exercise or one dimension of fitness at a time.

Track your efforts and accomplishments. When you've worked up to a half-hour walk or finally perfected an exercise, take note of it. Seeing a record of your progress is a motivation-booster that will help you focus on the next steps in your fitness journey. Some people like using a wearable fitness tracker or smartphone fitness app to keep them honest and monitor overall activity levels. Me, I'm old school. I simply use an old-fashioned desk calendar to record my workouts, walks, and yoga and Pilates sessions.

Listen to your body. Building a little bit of challenge into your workouts is good; that's how you can gradually extend your limits. But don't try to push *past* your limits by ignoring signals of fatigue or pain. If you're exhausted, you're much more likely to hurt yourself. And please don't ever, *ever* "push through" pain, no matter how macho it makes you feel. If a movement causes pain, it may be a sign that you're not doing the movement correctly, or perhaps shouldn't be doing it at all. When in doubt, err on the side of caution and consult a knowledgeable trainer or physical therapy professional.

Mix it up. Don't get stuck doing the same routine over and over—that only leads to boredom and diminishing returns. Doing a variety of movements and activities is the best way to keep things fresh while exercising all muscle groups.

START FROM WHERE YOU ARE AND CONCENTRATE ON MAKING SMALL, STEADY IMPROVEMENTS.

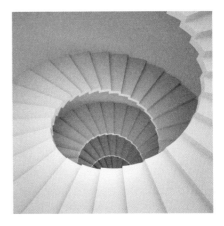

MAKE IT FUN

This is the ultimate secret of success. After all, the best exercises are the ones you will actually do. If you enjoy and want to do them, it's a win-win.

Find ways of moving that you enjoy. There are endless ways to be active. Try a spinning class, Pilates, or one of the increasingly popular movement classes designed for older adults. If gyms aren't your thing, exercise outdoors. Maybe you'd enjoy water aerobics, kayaking, or badminton. Try something new and see how it feels! Anything that gets you moving and uses a variety of muscles is worth checking out.

Use the whole world as your gym. Once you learn the principles of good posture and exercise form, you can begin applying them to everything you do. If you find yourself waiting in line at the post office, use that time to go up and down on your toes (a calf exercise) or practice standing up straight with your shoulders back. As you're putting groceries away, feel how far you can stretch, and then repeat that motion with the other side of your body. Not only will you get more out of doing routine chores, you'll begin to engage with your body on a whole new level.

**"MAKE IT FUN"
IS THE ULTIMATE
SECRET OF SUCCESS.
IF YOU ENJOY
EXERCISING—AND
WANT TO DO IT—
IT'S A WIN-WIN.**

Discover what inspires you. Maybe it's watching an Olympic skater or the stars of an NBA playoff game. It could be someone like Olga Kotelko, the 90-something track star whose amazing athletic ability is probed in the book *What Makes Olga Run?* Or it might be someone who's met a completely different type of challenge, like a disabled vet. Anything that makes you want to reach for your best self is an inspiration worth holding on to and revisiting whenever you need it.

Find the joy in every dimension of life. Becoming fit helped me recapture that feeling of "aliveness" that can so easily slip away as the years go by. I'm more in tune with the simple pleasures of the world around me. Now that I can move freely, I can experience and enjoy so much more. Everything about my life feels richer as a result.

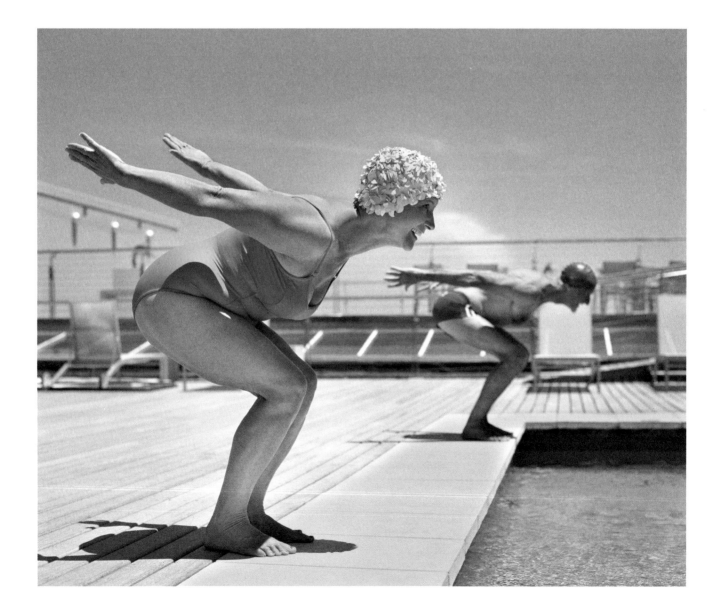

WHAT MOTIVATES YOU?

Experts agree that regular exercise is the best single prescription there is for successful aging.
So it's worth reflecting on what would motivate you to follow their advice. Think about the different ways
people you know have aged. Then think about how you want your life to be in 10, 15, or 20 years.
Go over the items you've marked "high" or "medium," and ask yourself:
Am I willing to invest an hour a day toward meeting those goals?

IMPORTANCE TO YOU

AS I GET OLDER, I WANT TO...	HIGH	MEDIUM	LOW
Look and feel younger than my years (and peers)			
Have more energy and vitality			
Stay active, travel, and do all the things I enjoy			
Be able to keep up with my children or grandchildren			
Keep playing my favorite sports			
Enjoy an active sex life			
Live in my own home as long as I possibly can			
Avoid becoming physically dependent upon anyone else			
Keep anxiety and depression at bay			
Prevent falls and injuries			
Lower my risks of heart disease, cancer, and stroke			
Reduce my day-to-day aches and pains			
Better manage a chronic health problem			
Reduce the number of prescription medications I must take			

THE POWER OF RITUAL

This chapter gives you a number of tips for making fitness a part of your life. But there is another technique that may be the most powerful of all. The secret is to turn your daily workout routine into a ritual. A ritual is a part of your day that feels so necessary and worthwhile that it's unquestioned...almost sacrosanct.

Think about the rituals that are already embedded in your daily life.
Having your morning coffee. Sharing a meal at the dinner table. Kissing your loved ones goodbye as they walk out the door. These aren't mere habits; they are interludes you take time to savor. They give shape to your life and help you move on to the next things in your day. They provide a calming sense of being anchored amid everything else going on around you. They turn the mundane details of life into special moments.

Gretchen Rubin, author of *The Happiness Project,* has made a study of ways we add satisfaction to our lives. As she writes in her latest book, *Better Than Before,* "a routine is a string of habits; a ritual is a habit charged with transcendent meaning."

So how can you make exercise transcendent?
The key word in the quote is "meaning." Once you have developed even a sketchy fitness routine, you can begin consciously connecting your exercise sessions with experiences, thoughts, and feelings that hold a deeper meaning for you.

When you operate in this spirit, exercising outdoors becomes a chance to reconnect with the beauty and majesty of nature. Think of your walks as welcome time for reflection if you're alone, or a time for sharing if you go with a friend. When you work out at the gym, take a moment to feel gratitude for the body that has kept you going all these years. And there's nothing like the burst of energy that follows a vigorous good workout to make you feel lucky to be alive!

If you are able to imbue your workouts with a sense of ritual, it becomes much easier to stick with the program. You no longer have to push yourself, because the ritual itself is a reward.

1 Assuming "more is better"
Studies show that most of the benefits from walking or other cardiovascular activity are gained in the first 30 minutes. Similarly, a well-designed hour-long workout should be enough to cover an appropriate range of exercises. Why wear yourself out for diminishing returns?

2 Thinking "I already know how to move"
Modern lifestyles work against the body's natural ways of moving. The vast majority of people need some training to change dysfunctional patterns of movement acquired over years of inactivity.

3 Not giving your body enough recovery time
Remember, exercise works by tearing down muscle fibers and stimulating the body to rebuild them. That takes time, especially when you get older. So don't do serious strength training with the same muscles two days in a row.

4 Getting distracted
Not only do lapses in attention undermine your progress, they can lead to strain or injury. When you work out, leave your cell phone in your locker and keep chatter to a minimum.

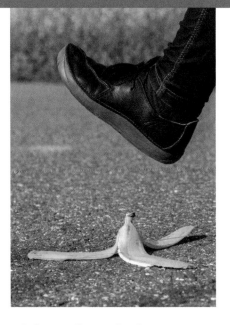

5 Demanding perfection
Don't expect to do an exercise flawlessly from the get-go. It can take time. In fact, the exercises you find hard to do with good form are probably the ones you most need to do. The goal is progress, not perfection.

6 Making excuses
The only one hurt by a failure to follow through is you. If you genuinely want to improve your fitness, you've got to take responsibility for your own efforts.

7 Being too impatient for rewards
It takes time and consistency for exercise to work its magic. Still, sports medicine experts say muscle strength can be improved in as little as eight weeks of resistance training, even in 90-year-olds.

Hang in there and you'll soon begin seeing results.

8 Letting your ego drive you
Succeeding at fitness isn't a competition to see how many repetitions you can do. That's strictly a numbers game. What makes the difference is what you can't see—namely, the quality and integrity of your effort. To get real results, focus on what's going on inside your body.

9 Allowing limitations to hold you back
Even professional athletes have weaknesses, past injuries, and other physical problems to cope with. With the right help, you can learn how to adapt and what to avoid so you can work out safely.

10 Not getting expert help
You wouldn't invest a huge sum of money without getting sound financial advice, would you? Is your health and quality of life any less important? It can take some searching to find people who are genuinely skilled physical training professionals (see Chapter 7 for some tips on that score). But when you do find the right trainer, it can be life-changing.

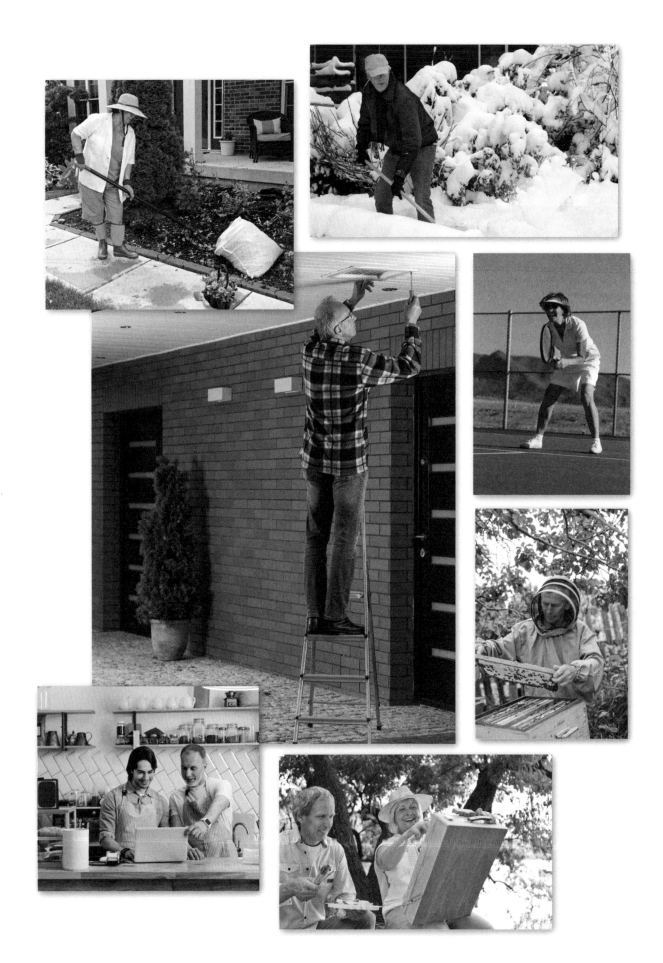

CHAPTER THREE

Functional Fitness
What It Means, Why You Need It

"SURE, I WORK OUT." This is what I often hear from friends when the conversation turns to fitness. I'm always interested in what other people, especially my contemporaries, are doing to stay in shape. When I ask them what regimens they're following, the answer is frequently something along the lines of, "I walk on the treadmill for half an hour at least two or three times a week." Or I might hear, "Every few days I go to the gym and do some machines." The women in our social circle often mention group classes like Zumba, yoga, or Pilates.

Those are all good forms of exercise, and they work fine as components of a fitness program. But are they enough to keep you moving comfortably through all your daily activities? Not even close—not if you subscribe to the notion of functional fitness. It's no coincidence that this phrase started cropping up a decade or so ago, about the time the first wave of baby boomers started noticing more aches and pains. Back then, working out was mostly geared to bodybuilding or slimming and toning. A lot of it was about looking youthful and sexy, having an impressive physique, or getting in shape for competitive sports.

IT'S ALL ABOUT TRAINING YOUR BODY TO MEET THE PHYSICAL DEMANDS OF DAILY LIFE.

A MORE PRACTICAL APPROACH

Functional fitness has a different and more practical purpose. It's about training your body to navigate all the daily activities of life without strain, pain, or injury. Walking, bending, reaching, climbing, lifting—such movements require multiple muscle groups working together in a sequential and coordinated way. To do them with ease, you need balanced muscular development, good core strength, and good posture as you move.

Until only recently, however, our country's fitness culture was dominated by a bodybuilding mentality that doesn't focus on the movements needed in daily living. Instead, it relies on machines and exercises that isolate muscles or

IN THIS CHAPTER

- *Why cardio machines aren't enough*

- *A different way to think about fitness*

- *What it takes to navigate a three-dimensional world*

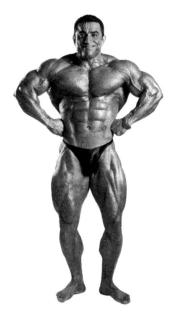

THE OLD CULTURE
OF BODYBUILDING
FOCUSED ON BUILDING
ISOLATED MUSCLES,
NOT IMPROVING
PHYSICAL FUNCTION.

muscle groups, aiming to strengthen them one at a time. It also tends to emphasize quantity rather than quality, measuring success by how much you've lifted and how many times. Functional concerns like range of motion and support for vulnerable joints get short shrift or are ignored altogether.

This is why knowledgeable trainers draw a distinction between being gym fit and functionally fit. Someone who's gym fit may be able to bench-press far more than his or her body weight, but still get injured while moving a piece of furniture or digging in the yard. Well aware of these hazards, professional sports teams now spend millions on coaches and facilities that center training on movements rather than muscles. Even LeBron James, one of the NBA's top players of all time, suffers from back problems and pulled muscles. Since 2009 his training has included yoga classes to help him stay flexible and avoid injuries. He's not alone; a growing number of professional football, basketball, baseball, and hockey teams have yoga instructors on their coaching rosters.

WHY VARIETY IS CRITICAL

Functional problems also arise if you depend mostly on a treadmill, elliptical trainer, or cross-trainer for exercise. Those kinds of machines can certainly raise your heart rate and, if used regularly, promote cardiovascular fitness. But they can lead to repetitive stress, and they alone won't make you functionally fit. That's because cardio machines keep you moving in just one plane, and most often, in one direction—forward. The same is true of walking, bicycling, and spinning.

In contrast, the movements that propel us through our everyday lives are three-dimensional and involve moving in all three spatial planes—the vertical plane (forward and backward), the horizontal plane (from side to side), and in rotation. They also require different types of movements at the body's joints. (See page 56, "The Dynamics of Movement," for more on these concepts.)

If functional fitness is what you're after, a balanced program is the way to get there. By that, I mean a program that addresses all five facets of fitness:

- *Core stability and strength*

- *Flexibility*

- *Balance*

- *Muscular strength*

- *Cardiovascular endurance*

If that sounds overwhelming, don't worry. Many of the basic exercises I recommend later in this book will serve two or more objectives at once. That's one reason why it only makes sense to build workouts around whole-body movements. Functional training borrows from a variety of approaches and disciplines, including yoga, Pilates, dance, and physical therapy as well as resistance training. Once you understand what it's about, you'll see it doesn't have to be complicated. You will also be able to work its principles into your daily chores and activities, so your training extends into everything you do.

A MIND-SET THAT FITS

It's striking to look back and realize how much the thinking on fitness has evolved. Those of us born between World War II and the mid-1960s came of age at a time when working out was mainly for athletes and bodybuilders. It wasn't until the 1970s that the fitness boom took hold, as millions of Americans began jogging, distance running, and doing Jazzercize. And it wasn't until well after 1972, when Congress passed Title IX, the federal law prohibiting gender discrimination in public education, that athletic programs for girls began to blossom. So it's not surprising that many in my generation still see aging as inexorable and working out as something for muscleheads.

But we're also ideally positioned to bring a new fitness paradigm to the fore. In our time we've witnessed an astonishing stream of scientific breakthroughs. We now know that exercise affects our bodies at a deep, molecular level, and that the aging process is more malleable than previously thought. We've also seen an explosion of health clubs, home fitness devices, and training methods (not to mention more than 30 years of Jane Fonda workout videos).

Now we are at the age where ease of movement is more important than having six-pack abs and "jacked" muscles—and we've got strength in numbers. Don't think the fitness industry hasn't noticed. Gym memberships used to be concentrated in the 18-to-34 age group. These days, much of their growth is coming from the 50-and-over demographic. Movement classes for older adults are springing up at community centers and YMCAs all across the country, and a growing number of gyms and trainers specialize in programs tailored to an aging population.

FUNCTIONAL TRAINING EMPHASIZES WHOLE-BODY MOVEMENTS AND ADDRESSES ALL FIVE FACETS OF FITNESS.

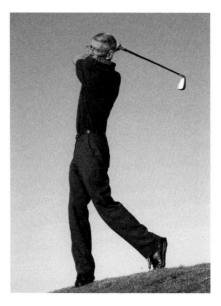

Beyond that, fitness-minded people of all ages are moving toward exercises that use your own body weight for resistance rather than relying solely on barbells or traditional machines. In fact, the American College of Sports Medicine recently ranked bodyweight training as a top fitness trend.

This is why I'm convinced that functional fitness is the wave of the future. The old gym culture's focus on appearance rather than function no longer fits the baby boomer generation. After all, bulging biceps don't do a guy much good if he can't climb stairs without stabbing pain in his knees. By the same token, being model-slim doesn't mean a woman can lift her grandchild from a stroller without throwing out her back.

So don't be intimidated if you walk into a gym and see a lot of members who look like they're auditioning to play the Incredible Hulk or Wonder Woman. You'll know that you are on a different path—one with its own goals, challenges, and rewards. If the contrast is distracting, you can always seek out another gym, trainer, or fitness studio that's more attuned to the functional fitness idea. With the program later in this book, you can also design a customized fitness regimen for working out at home, outdoors, in the gym, or all of the above. Options abound, and they're expanding every day.

Our generation radically changed the culture of America. Now we're changing the culture of fitness, too.

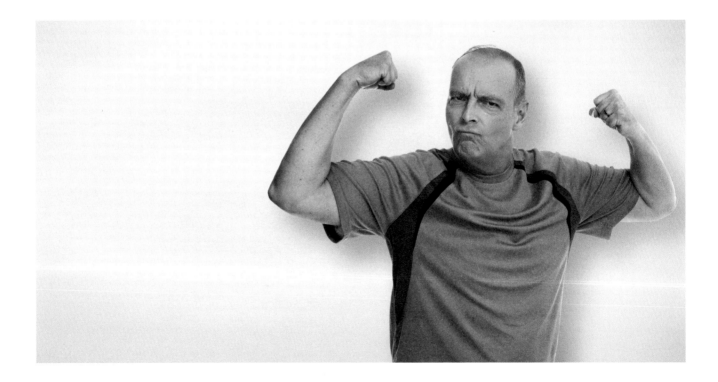

HOW THE FITNESS PARADIGM IS SHIFTING

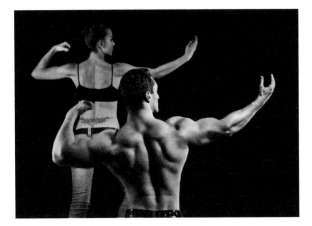 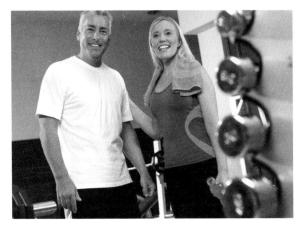

	OUT WITH THE OLD	IN WITH THE NEW
GOALS	• Bodybuilding (mainly for men) • Slimming/toning (mainly for women)	• Functional fitness for both genders
TRAINING	• One-dimensional—usually strength or cardio	• Across all five facets of fitness
CENTERED ON	• Muscle-isolating exercises involving a single joint	• Multi-joint or whole-body exercises
RELIES ON	• Machines and barbells	• Light dumbbells, cables, bodyweight resistance
FOCUS ON	• Quantity—how much weight; how many repetitions	• Quality of effort and form
VALUES	• Muscular strength, size and definition	• Agility and ease of motion
COMPETITION	• To be the strongest or best looking	• Only with yourself
STRIVES FOR	• Looking good	• Feeling good
DRIVEN BY	• Vanity and ego	• Quality of life

ATTITUDE
MAKES ALL THE DIFFERENCE

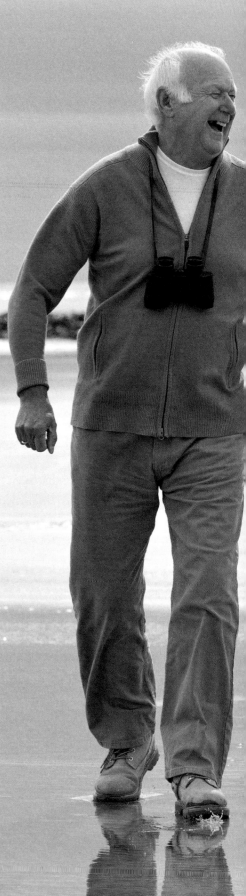

AS I'VE LEARNED FIRSTHAND, aging isn't a linear process. You can go along for months and years, feeling pretty much like the same person you always did, despite the wrinkles here and there. And then, one day, something shifts. Maybe you notice a twinge or pain you never felt before. Or the flight of steps you could scale in a bound suddenly feels like your personal Everest. With a shock, you hear that little voice inside saying, "Uh-oh! I'm OLD." And you get the feeling that life is all downhill from here on in.

Maybe that hasn't happened to you yet, even if you're past 65 or 70. But trust me...sooner or later, it will. Then those elderly jokes start to have a different ring to them. ("You know you're getting old when all the names in your little black book have 'M.D.' after them.")

Realizing that you've arrived at a new and different stage in life isn't necessarily a bad thing. But then what?

On one hand, acknowledging physical changes that come with age is vital if you want to keep from injuring yourself. It can also bring you newfound peace of mind. As environmental activist Dominique Browning wrote in a wonderful *New York Times* essay titled "I'm Too Old for This," accepting where you are in life can also be "profoundly liberating," freeing you from youthful insecurities about not measuring up when you look in the mirror.

At the same time, deciding you want to get fitter and stave off disability is liberating in a different way, and empowering, too. People who approach aging with a positive outlook take better care of themselves and tend to be in better shape, longitudinal studies show. They also live an average of 7.5 years longer than those who equate age with infirmity, even after other health factors are taken into account.

In other words, what aging is like for you has a lot to do with your attitude about the process. Said Pablo Picasso, who reached the age of 91, "Youth has no age."

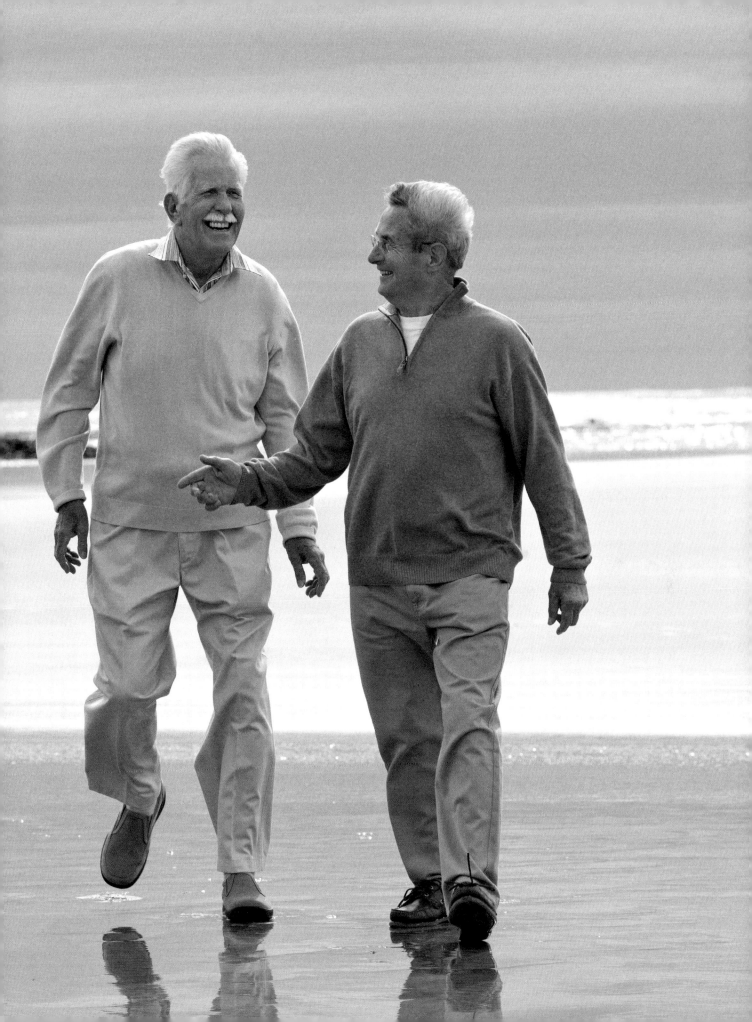

THE DYNAMICS OF
MOVEMENT

While you could spend a lifetime studying biomechanics, there's no need to get overwhelmed at the outset of your fitness journey. Still, being familiar with a few basic concepts — like moving in all three planes of motion— will help you understand what different exercises are designed to do and why it's important to do varied types of movements. The lunge is an ideal example because it's an exercise that can be done in all three planes. These concepts will also come into play as we talk about designing and customizing your workout in later chapters.

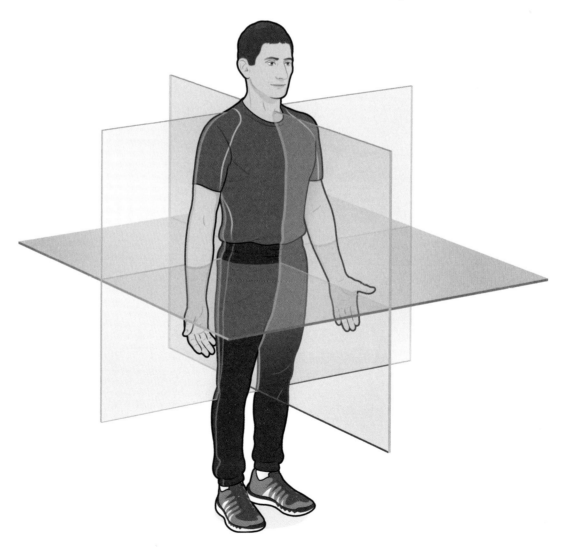

THREE PLANES OF MOTION

Sagittal Plane *Divides the body into left/right*

Movements along this plane propel the body forward or backward, as when we're walking, running, or biking, or involve folding movements, such as squatting or bending over.

Frontal Plane *Divides the body into front/back*

Motions along this plane go out to the side (which is why the "frontal" label can be confusing). Examples include side lunges and jumping jacks.

Transverse Plane *Divides the body into top/bottom*

Whenever we rotate horizontally or twist from the spine—for example, turning to reach or look behind us—we are moving in the transverse plane. Many sports call for transverse movements; think of swinging a baseball bat, tennis racket, or golf club. Many people have limited range of movement in this plane and tend to avoid rotational movements. For them, it's especially important to do some stretches and exercises that open up the hips and shoulders and restore movement around the spine.

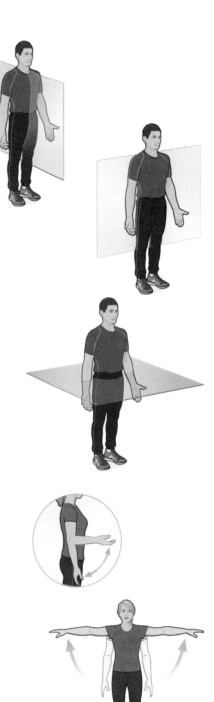

OTHER CONCEPTS TO KNOW

Extension vs. Flexion These movements affect the angle between two adjacent body parts. Flexion decreases that angle, as when you bend your elbow, squat, or sit down. Extension is a movement that straightens the body and increases the angle between body parts.

Internal vs. External Rotation Our major joints, such as hips and shoulders, can rotate both internally (down and forward, or toward the middle of the body) and externally (up and outward, or away from the middle of the body). Most of us need to work more on moving outward and upward because gravity and our habits of sitting tend to draw us downward and inward. *(Not pictured.)*

Abduction vs. Adduction These terms describe movement of the limb or other body parts away from one of the center lines of the body (abduction) or toward the center line (adduction). These movements can be vertical (as in the example shown), or horizontal, or combined with internal or external rotation. Most of us generally move in a range fairly close to our midlines.

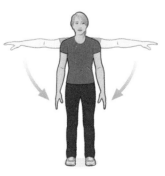

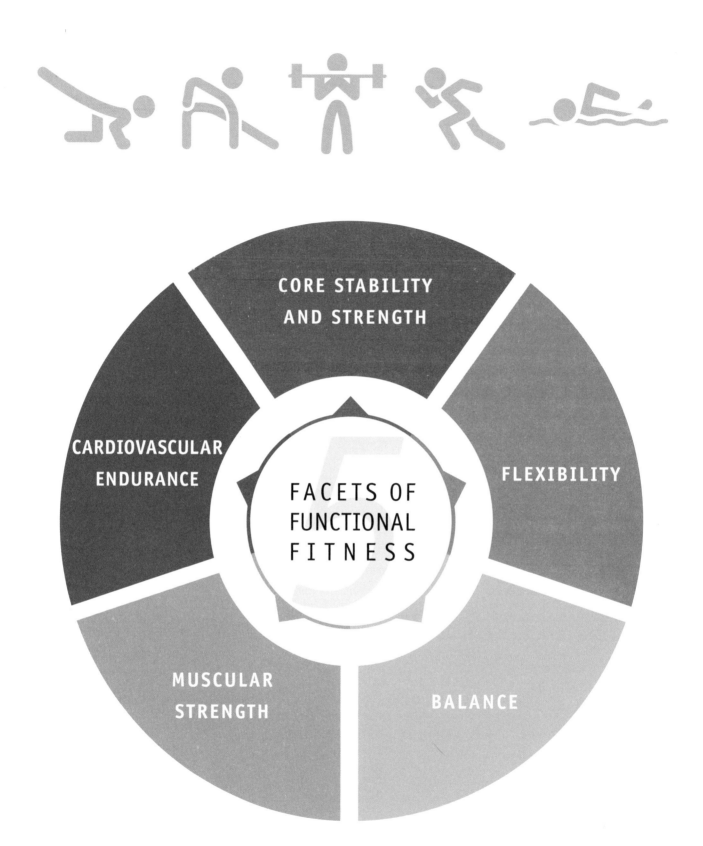

CHAPTER FOUR

5 Facets of Functional Fitness

To Be Fit, You Need a Program as Multidimensional as Your Body

EVERY DAY you count on your body to do many different things. It's an amazingly capable and protean machine—a marvel of bioengineering. The human body is equipped to move, bend, stretch, climb, jump, and manipulate objects both large and small. It can also adapt to its surroundings, grow new cells, ward off foreign invaders, and even heal itself. So doesn't it stand to reason that your body's needs for activity and exercise are multidimensional, too?

Yet I keep meeting people who exercise solely by doing slow cardio on a treadmill or cross-trainer, and then wonder why they're not getting noticeably stronger and leaner. Others swear by yoga as their all-around fitness solution. Although a tremendously beneficial discipline with millions of devotees, yoga alone won't make you fit, either. Nor will tennis or kickboxing or just about any other single activity I can think of.

Doing just one kind of exercise won't prevent or reverse the effects of aging in all the ways that you need to get or stay fit. A one-track approach is especially problematic when you're older. Too much of the same kind of motion can overtax muscles and joints, putting you at risk of repetitive stress injuries. A one-dimensional routine also leaves some parts of your body unchallenged, leading to imbalances and weaknesses. Besides, it gets boring!

This chapter will make it clear why the principle of diversification, that core tenet of Investing 101, applies to fitness, too. The American College of Sports Medicine and the American Heart Association agree: their current fitness guidelines for adults over 65 (and those 50 to 64 with chronic health issues) explicitly call for training programs with a mix of strength building, flexibility, and balance, as well as aerobic activities. But don't worry! A more varied fitness program doesn't necessarily translate into a bigger time commitment. In fact, understanding the five facets of fitness will help you get more rewards from the time you devote to fitness. With the right mix of activities, and

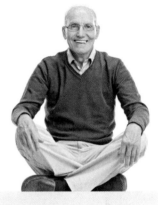

IN THIS CHAPTER

- *How each of the five facets of fitness contributes to well-being*

- *Why we get progressively stiffer and tighter with age—and what you can do about it*

- *How to lower your risk of falling*

- *The best defenses against back pain*

- *How strength training can help you lose weight*

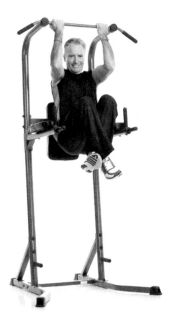

enough focus and intensity, you can target your real fitness issues and get measurable, visible results in one hour a day.

CORE STABILITY AND STRENGTH

Before I got the fitness bug, I had no idea what the body's "core" even meant; it sounded like a buzzword. But I soon learned why core stability and strength are critical if you want to stay active and keep your quality of life as you age.

People often think of the core as equivalent to the abs, that "six-pack" workout magazines are always talking about. In fact, your core encompasses all the muscles of your torso—not just your abdominals, but also your upper and lower back and glutes (buttocks). The core extends into your hips and your thigh muscles (front, back, outer, and inner), which support and assist your body's large muscles as you walk, lift, or squat. Finally, there are the obliques, the muscles that run diagonally along both sides of your midsection and are vital to any twisting or rotating movement.

It's clear that your core is the bridge between your upper and lower body. But its role in your daily life goes far beyond that. The strong muscles of the core provide the force that lets you stand up straight, walk down the street, pick up a bag of groceries, or swing a golf club.

In essence, your core muscles are your body's stability and power center. The stabilizers are the muscles that attach to the spine and support its movements; they help you stay balanced and in control as you move. The movers are the large muscles that move your body through all three planes of motion, often working together with or in support of other muscles.

When you think about it, most of the movements we make begin near the center of the body and move outward. That's why you need strong core muscles at any age. They provide the base of support and power for just about everything you do. Let the force be with you!

WHY CORE STRENGTH IS SO IMPORTANT

Support every move. A strong core supports your spine, so your entire body is more structurally sound whether you are standing, moving, turning, or lifting. Having weak core muscles is the main reason why so many older people have trouble with movements like getting in and out of chairs. If you can't sit down and get up from a dining room chair without using your arms, take it as a sign that your core needs work.

Have a pain-free back. It's estimated that 80 percent of Americans suffer from lower back pain at some point in their lives, most often without knowing the source of the problem. Moreover, studies suggest that treatments such as cortisone injections have fewer lasting benefits than movement-based strategies like walking and yoga. A strong core is vital to support your spine and keep it properly aligned in its natural "S-curve" shape as you move. Without that support, you have less stability and control in your movements, increasing the likelihood that you will "tweak" or throw out your back. A focus on core exercises certainly paid off for me. Because of my history of back injuries, I spent a good 25 to 30 percent of every workout on core exercises when I first started working out. After a year of stretching tight muscles and strengthening my core, I was virtually pain-free.

Alleviate stress on joints. If your core is weak, or if you tend to sit, stand, or move without engaging those muscles, your bones and joints have to handle more of the load.

Help prevent falls. A strong core will help you stay balanced and in control of your movements. It will also increase your flexibility and range of motion as you move, another line of defense against falls.

Improve posture and breathing. It takes good core muscles to stand up straight, and standing up straight will help strengthen core muscles—a classic "virtuous circle." Better posture will lower your risk of herniated disks and degeneration of the vertebrae, orthopedists say.

ABOUT 80% OF AMERICANS SUFFER WITH LOWER BACK PAIN AT SOME POINT IN THEIR LIVES.

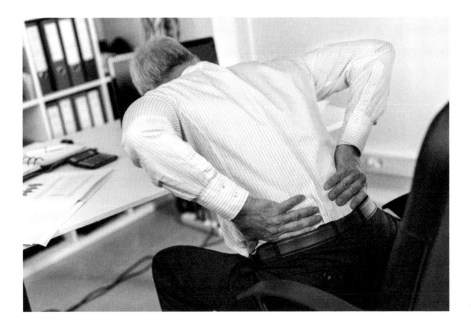

YOUR CORE MUSCLES
ARE YOUR BODY'S
STABILITY AND
POWER CENTER.

WHAT TO DO

Concentrate on whole-body exercises. Go for movements that engage multiple core muscles and tend to mimic movements we do in real life. They will strengthen your core more efficiently, and in a more balanced way, than exercises that isolate just one part of the core, like crunches. The basic exercises I recommend in Chapter 7 include some that are especially beneficial for the core, including the plank, the squat, and variations of the push-up. For all-around core-strengthening, it's important to include vertical core exercises—ones you do standing up—as well as exercises done on a mat.

Skip the crunches and sit-ups. What's the one exercise to do for your abdominals? If you're like most people, you probably thought first of sit-ups or crunches. The trouble is, both exercises put stress on your spine and neck, especially if you're not doing them perfectly. There are many other core exercises that are easy to do safely and have a much better payoff. Why take the risk?

Learn the pelvic tuck. This is an important move to learn because most of us walk around with our backbones out of alignment. Also known as the pelvic tilt, it's a small, subtle move, but one that's vital to know if you want to protect your spine and use the right muscles as you move. In essence, the pelvic tuck involves tightening your gluteal muscles as though you're pulling your pelvis

CORE MUSCLES

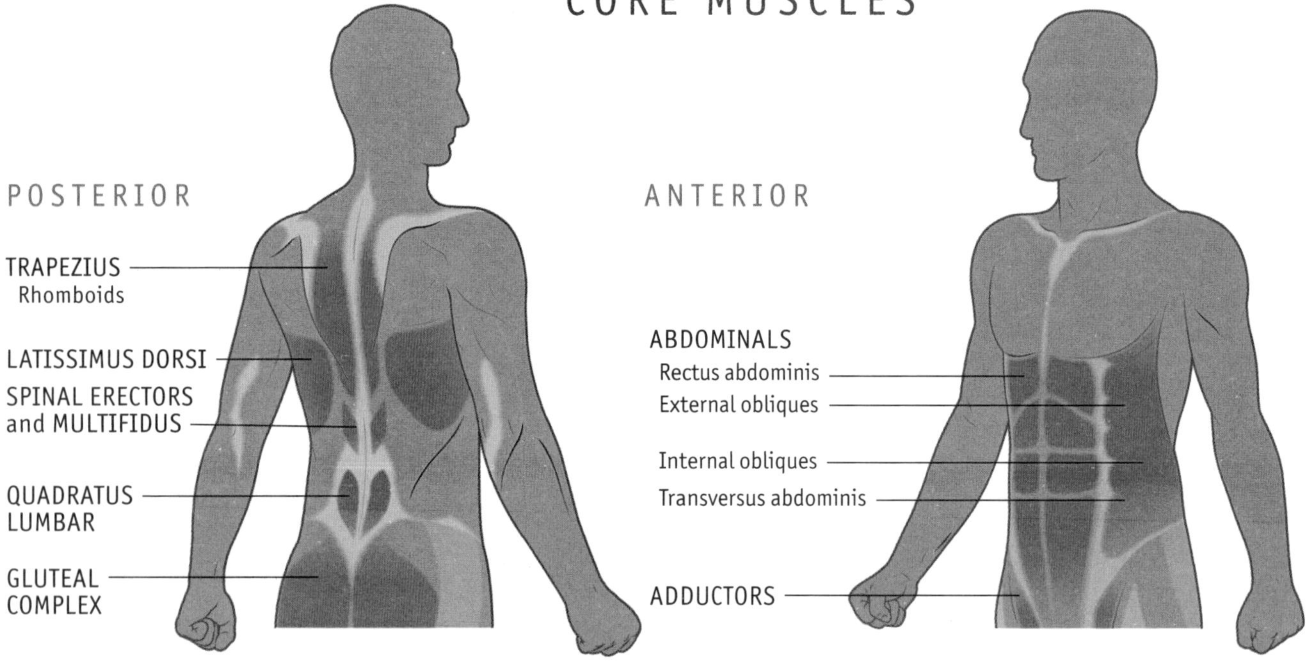

POSTERIOR

TRAPEZIUS
Rhomboids

LATISSIMUS DORSI

SPINAL ERECTORS
and MULTIFIDUS

QUADRATUS
LUMBAR

GLUTEAL
COMPLEX

ANTERIOR

ABDOMINALS
Rectus abdominis
External obliques

Internal obliques
Transversus abdominis

ADDUCTORS

up toward your belly button, so you move your spine into a neutral, properly aligned position. The pelvic tilt (also known as "neutral spine") is described more fully in the section on posture in Chapter 6. Give it a try and you'll feel the difference.

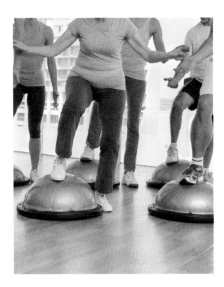

Don't neglect your back muscles. Many people think a strong core comes from focusing on your abdominals, but that approach may do more harm than good. Having strong abs but weak back muscles, or the reverse, is a recipe for lower back trouble.

Engage your core throughout the day. Try this: stand as straight and tall as you can, with your chest held high and shoulders back. Do you feel the tautness in your abdominals, back, gluteal muscles, and upper thighs? Your muscles are experiencing static stress, meaning they are contracting involuntarily, even though your body isn't moving. That's a good kind of stress, because it helps strengthen muscles and builds endurance. In short, it counts as exercise! This is one more way good posture pays off. It lets you exercise your core whenever you stand, walk, and move around. You can apply the same principle while sitting if you move your bottom toward the edge of your chair and use your muscles, rather than the furniture, to hold your body upright. Using a Swiss ball in place of a chair, as I now do in my home office, is a great strategy for keeping your core engaged.

Do Pilates, yoga, or both. A Pilates class is a terrific core-strengthener because it concentrates on movements that originate from the center of your body. Yoga can also do more for core muscles than you think; many of the postures build core strength and stability as you learn to achieve and hold them.

ADVANCED: Do exercises on unstable surfaces. Basic exercises like a plank, a push-up, or a squat do a lot more for core muscles if you do them on an unstable surface like a Bosu (an inflated half sphere, which you'll find in any well-equipped gym) or a Swiss ball. However, I'd advise that you try this only with the help of a knowledgeable trainer—do not attempt it alone.

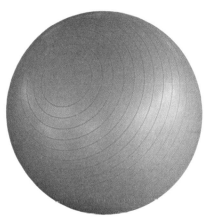

SWISS BALL

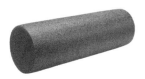

FOAM ROLLER

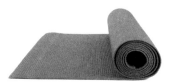

EXERCISE/YOGA MAT

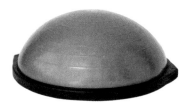

BOSU

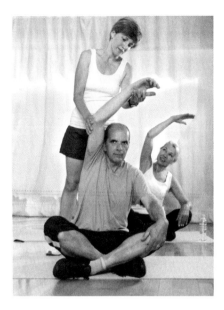

IF YOU DON'T
WORK ON IT,
YOUR RANGE OF
MOTION ONLY
GETS WORSE.

FLEXIBILITY

Are you bothered by aches and pains? Feel stiff and creaky, especially when you first get up from your chair or a night's sleep? A lack of flexibility could be the culprit.

Flexibility means your ability to carry a movement through its entire range of motion. Also known as limberness, it depends on the mobility of your joints, the length of your muscles, and the elasticity of your tendons, ligaments, and connective tissue.

It's an aspect of fitness that is widely underrated, even by people who are active and strong. In my estimation, a lack of flexibility is responsible for perhaps 80 percent of the typical aches and pains of aging. And it's a problem that only gets worse with age.

If you don't make a point of moving your muscles and joints through their full range of motion, over time your body becomes progressively tighter. By degrees, you lose the ability to stand up straight, bend over and touch your toes, or turn and look behind you. Getting in or out of a car becomes more difficult. It's harder to pull a sweater over your head. And you begin developing that stooped, hunched-over posture that shouts, "I'm old!" It's a vicious circle: the more restricted your movements, the less you're doing to preserve your mobility. As one wise woman in her eighties put it: "If you rest, you rust."

Why are flexibility problems virtually universal among the older crowd? Not to harp on the subject, but sitting is one big reason. If you spend too much time in chairs, then your hamstrings, the large muscles at the back of your thighs, no longer fully extend. Soon your hips are tight and permanently flexed, affecting how you stand and walk. It took me years to discover that tight hips were a root cause of my excruciating back pain! Poor posture, rounded shoulders, tight calves and ankles, and limited rotation of the torso are all part of the syndrome. People with imbalanced muscular development, like many bodybuilders, are prone to flexibility problems, too.

WHY FLEXIBILITY IS SO IMPORTANT

Avoid pain and injury. Now I understand why I kept throwing out my back. If some muscles and joints are inflexible, your movements will be limited or distorted. Some muscle groups may shut down, while others get overloaded as they're forced to pitch in and take up the slack. If muscles and joints have to move in ways the body isn't designed to do, you will have aches and soreness, if not an acute or chronic injury.

Protect tendons and ligaments. Overuse or misuse of muscles can lead to tendonitis, a painful inflammation of the bands of tissue that connect muscles to bones. One version is popularly known as "tennis elbow," but tendonitis can also occur in shoulders, knees, wrists, heels—anywhere tendons are found in the body. You can also strain the ligaments that connect one bone to another, an injury that can take weeks or months to heal.

Lower risks of a devastating fall. Experts say a lack of flexibility is a major factor contributing to falls. The more flexible you are, the better your ability to react to an unexpected bump or obstacle, and to recover if you do begin to lose your balance.

Get through your day without mishap. Reaching for something, doing chores around the house, raking in the yard—even simple tasks become more difficult and more likely to cause injuries if your movements are restricted by a lack of flexibility.

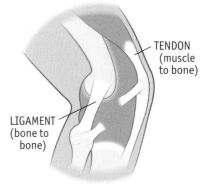

TENDON
(muscle
to bone)

LIGAMENT
(bone to
bone)

WHAT TO DO

Stretch. Stretching doesn't require a lot of time, but it's absolutely essential if you want to preserve or regain your flexibility. That's why the first step in the fitness program outlined in this book is stretching on a regular basis—a full session at least three times a week, and a few minutes when you're going out for a walk or whenever you feel tight (see Chapter 5). Some people like to stretch first thing in the morning to help them get ready for the day. Stretching doesn't have to be burdensome; you can break it up into multiple sessions and even do some stretches while you watch the news, talk on the phone, or wait in line. Truthfully, I was skeptical at first. But it's ended up making a huge difference in my workouts and my daily life—I feel so much better. Try it and you'll see!

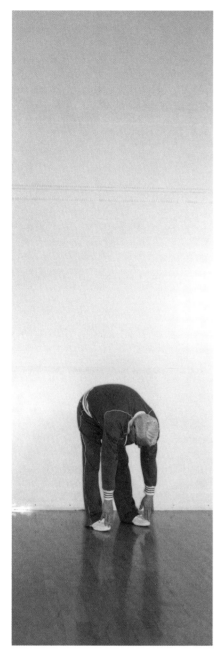

Use a foam roller. The foam roller has become my new best friend; I've found nothing that does more to release muscle tightness and gently break up knotted areas. Five minutes of foam rolling is always, **_always_** part of my workout. Rollers are inexpensive and easily tucked into your closet at home.

Be aware of your patterns of movement. If you think about range of motion as you move through your day, you'll find many ways to work on flexibility. Don't avoid bending over; embrace it as an easy way to exercise. Use every physical chore as an opportunity to move and stretch. (See Chapter 7 for tips on movement form; they will help you improve your functionality even if you don't work out in a gym.)

Make sure your workouts cover a variety of muscle groups. If you develop one muscle group and ignore the opposing one, the resulting imbalance could cause functional problems and continuing pain.

Take a yoga or Pilates class. Flexibility is at the core of these two disciplines, and they can be life-changing for people with tight muscles or stress-related muscular tension. They can also improve breathing, strength, and mindfulness.

See a good physical therapist. If chronic pain or movement issues are interfering with your life, it's worth getting professional help. A movement expert can diagnose what's causing your problems and give you the right exercises to prevent or ease them. Your doctor or trainer should be able to refer you to a credentialed PT.

Get regular deep-tissue massages. It may sound like a luxury, but massage from a skilled bodyworker can be highly therapeutic. Besides easing tightness in muscles, connective tissues, tendons, ligaments, and joints, massage therapy can stimulate blood flow and ease stress. Use your network to find the best massage therapist in your area, and book a session at least once a month.

IF BENDING OVER IS DIFFICULT, DON'T AVOID IT! TAKE IT AS A SIGNAL THAT'S WHAT YOUR BODY NEEDS TO DO.

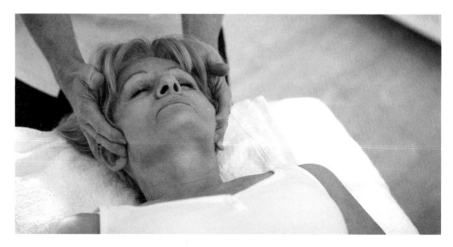

TEST YOUR FLEXIBILITY A = Excellent, B = Good, C = Needs work

Flexibility measures the extent to which we can stretch a static muscle. Mobility involves flexibility and adds a movement component, that is, range of motion in more than one plane. Both are important and play a crucial role in most everything we do, from tying our shoes to the way in which we walk. Circle the statements below that apply to you and see how your ratings stack up. If you tend to be stiff, you may want to spend a minute or two gently moving your body to warm up first.

Reach for Your Toes

Stand with your feet hip distance apart, arms hanging at your side and legs straight (a little flex in the knees is okay, but just a little). Bend from the hips and let your arms fall.

- A   I can put my palms on the floor.
- B   My fingers can touch the floor.
- C   My fingers are two inches or more from touching the floor.

Turn Your Head

In a standing or sitting position, raise your chin and move it first to the left and then to the right, gazing over your shoulder.

- A   I was able to move my head with ease and look behind me.
- B   One side was notably stiffer than the other (notice which one).
- C   I had to move my shoulders and upper body to see behind me.

The Back Scratch Test

Raise and bend one arm, drop your hand behind your back and bend your other arm up to reach behind your back. Try to meet the fingers on both hands. Repeat on the opposite side. Note the differences on each side.

- A   I was able to touch fingers on both hands.
- B   One side was notably more flexible than the other (notice which one).
- C   No chance. My fingers might as well have been in different countries.

Test Your Hip Mobility

1 Lying down on a flat surface, bend your knees and bring them to your chest, hugging them with both arms.
- A   I was able to bend both knees, bring them to my chest, and keep my lower back on the floor.
- B   I couldn't get my knees to my chest without raising my lower back from the surface.

2 Again, lying flat on your back, bend and bring one knee to your chest, hug it with both arms and hold for ten seconds. Repeat with the other leg. Note how your knees track. They should go straight into your chest, not off to the side.
- A   I could bring both knees (independently) to my chest while keeping my lower back on the ground.
- B   I could bring both knees up, but one knee or the other (or both) went out to the side.
- C   I could bring both knees up, but I was not able to keep my lower back on the surface.

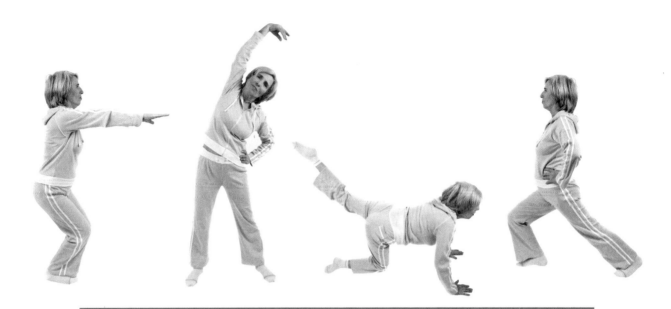

WHY WE LOSE FLEXIBILITY

IT'S NOT HARD TO UNDERSTAND why flexibility declines with the passing years. When muscles and tendons are relaxed, they are crinkled like an accordion. If not stretched often or far enough, they become chronically shortened and tight. Tightness can also be caused by muscular tension from stress, hard physical work, or any habitual activity that involves a limited range of motion (like running). Muscles that spend most of their time contracted rather than extended commonly develop *adhesions*—knots of muscle fibers that become stuck together and can cause pain.

Another important part of this picture is a little-known structure called *fascia*—the tough, springy connective tissue found throughout the body. Your fascia (the lighter areas in the illustration) wraps around and through all your muscles and tendons, giving them their shape and suppleness. If not continually stretched by frequent, varied movement, fascial tissues lose

elasticity and grow brittle. As they lose resilience, they begin to constrict your movements—imagine wearing an old sweater that keeps shrinking and getting tighter. The intertwining nature of the fascia is one reason why tightness or injury in one area of your body can affect other areas you might think are unrelated.

To see an example of "range of motion" in action, extend your arm as far as you can, keeping your palm facing up and your elbow straight; now bend at the elbow and touch your shoulder. If you can do that, you have a full range of motion for that particular movement. But realize that one motion isn't enough to gauge your flexibility; people are typically more flexible in some parts of the body than others. It's also true that women are generally more flexible than men. Not only do women tend to have longer muscles, they also benefit from female hormones that make connective tissue looser and childbirth easier.

BALANCE

Balance is a subject often neglected by even the most ardent fitness buffs. It's another one of those physical abilities we take for granted—until, that is, we feel it almost literally slipping away. When you're five years old, that dizzy, disoriented feeling you get from spinning in a circle is fun. When you're middle-aged or older, being unsteady on your feet can turn ordinary activities like getting dressed or navigating a flight of stairs into dangerous hurdles. The statistics are stark: each year one in three Americans over 65 takes a tumble, and the consequences can be disastrous or even fatal.

Few of us can expect to reach old age without experiencing some loss in our sense of balance; it's a normal consequence of aging. Balance issues can also be caused or exacerbated by other factors such as inner ear infections, low blood pressure, certain medications, and some chronic diseases.

But did you know that our ability to balance begins to weaken not in middle age, as you might expect, but when we are in our twenties? This is a huge reality check! Most of us go on for decades assuming that our bodies will do their balancing act without our even having to think about it. In truth, we need to start being more conscious of balance many years before the Medicare card arrives.

Balance turns out to be a complex and fine-tuned system that depends on a combination of physical abilities. At the top of the list is your *proprioception*— your body's ability to know where it is in space and react, consciously or unconsciously, to that stimulation. Can you close your eyes and still put your finger on your nose? That's an example of your proprioception in action.

Proprioception has three main sensory inputs:

- **Your vision.** This is why it is much harder to balance with your eyes closed.

- **Specialized sensory receptors.** Called proprioceptors, these sense movement in your muscles, tendons, and ligaments. Your feet, spine, and upper neck are densely packed with these sensors, but they are also found throughout the soft tissues of the body.

- **The vestibular system of the inner ear.** Tiny hairs in its semicircular canals transmit information on gravity and motion to your brain.

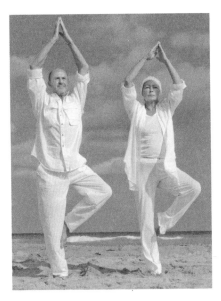

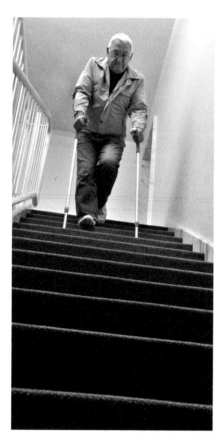

FEAR OF FALLING
CAN BE A BIG
PROBLEM IN ITSELF.

All of these senses tend to diminish with age, as do the agility, coordination, and muscular strength you must also have in order to maintain your balance.

Injuries can also impair balance by damaging ligaments and the neuroreceptors in joints. Ankle sprains are especially common and often lead to chronic instability in this part of the body, which happens to be one that exercise programs often overlook. So it's no wonder that falls are epidemic among the older crowd! Weakened proprioception can also be a cause of poor posture and chronic muscle and joint pain.

The good news is some simple exercises can help preserve and even restore your sense of balance if you do them regularly. Studies show that exercise can also reduce the odds of being seriously injured if you do fall. It's important to realize that balance involves two kinds of motor skills. Standing still requires static balance, while it takes dynamic balance to walk or climb stairs. Exercise can help by increasing strength of the ankle, knee, and hip muscles; by strengthening the vestibular system; or both.

You don't need any special devices or skills to get started. Your most important piece of equipment is the floor! Research suggests, however, that an integrated approach that also builds muscle strength, coordination, and flexibility is even more effective than balance training alone. The program in this book is designed to cover all those bases. Like so many other aspects of fitness, maintaining your balance is ultimately a whole-body challenge.

WHY BALANCE IS SO IMPORTANT

Falls can be devastating. More than 13 million Americans reported fall-related injuries in 2010, and the results were especially dire for those over 65. Falls left Americans in that age group with 2.5 million injuries bad enough to send them to the emergency room, 250,000 hip fractures, and more than 25,000 deaths, due mostly to traumatic brain injuries. In fact, falls account for three-fourths of accidental deaths among people in this age group. Falls are especially serious for those who take certain medications, like blood thinners. ***Any older person who falls and hits his or her head should see a doctor immediately.***

The problem only gets worse if ignored. Once you've experienced a fall, your chances of falling again are doubled, according to the Centers for Disease Control and Prevention (CDC). The fear of falling can be a big problem in itself. People who are afraid of losing their footing become less active and even weaker—a vicious cycle that only further increases their chances of falling again.

WHAT TO DO

Get in the habit of moving more mindfully. When you're young, you don't have to think much about balance. But when you're older and proprioceptive systems are weakened, you need to pay attention as you move and be especially aware of where you are placing your feet. It's also important to avoid multitasking and other distractions when you're in motion. A lapse of even a second or two may be enough to send you tumbling! See Chapter 5 for more on body awareness and how you can strengthen it. While you're at it, take some time to eliminate any hazards in your surroundings and get rid of footwear that could cause you to stumble.

Build simple, all-around balance exercises into your day. Stand on one foot while you brush your teeth, talk on the phone, or wash dishes. Get dressed standing up, so that you are standing on one foot as you put on your pants or shoes. Walk heel-to-toe with one foot directly in front of the other. Even two or three minutes a day of such moves will help fine-tune your balance over time.

Incorporate balance into your workouts. See the exercises in the following chapters for some candidates. It also makes sense to include exercises specifically designed to strengthen areas of past injury or weakness, especially the ankle if you've ever had a sprain. Ask a physical therapist or consult the American Physical Therapy Association's excellent *Book of Body Maintenance and Repair*.

Take up tai chi or yoga. While tai chi is a surprisingly good all-around workout, its slow, precise movements are ideal for improving balance, mindfulness, and confidence as you move. One study found that tai chi reduced falls in seniors by up to 45 percent. Yoga is also good for balance as well as flexibility.

ADVANCED: Use stability devices. Once you are practiced at working out, you can add a balance dimension to exercises by doing them on an unstable surface. You might start with the simplest versions, like the elliptical foam pads or an air-filled disk, and work up to devices like a wobble board or the Bosu. Any well-equipped gym should have some of these devices, which can be used for a variety of standing, kneeling, sitting, and push-up exercises. Some are inexpensive enough to have at home, or you can use a pillow.

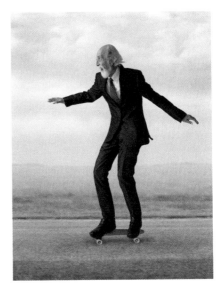

NOW *THAT'S* BALANCE!

TEST YOUR BALANCE   A = Excellent, B = Good, C = Needs work

Stand with Your Eyes Closed

Stand with your feet together and close your eyes. Count to ten.

- A I was able to stand still during the whole ten seconds.
- B I started to sway slightly over the course of the test.
- C I had to put a foot out to keep from toppling over.

One-Legged Stand

Before you begin this test, be sure to have something stable nearby to grab (just in case). Stand with your feet hip-distance apart; then lift one foot. Count to 30. Repeat with the other leg.

- A I was able to do this with no problem.
- B I was more successful with one leg than the other (note which one).
- C I faltered and swayed.

SIGNS OF TROUBLE

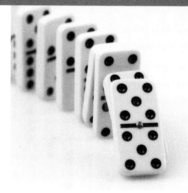

DON'T WAIT FOR A FALL to push you into doing something! If you've noticed any of the following problems, you should see your doctor for testing in addition to exploring some balance-oriented exercises. Balance disorders can be caused by inner ear, central nervous system, cardiovascular, or vision problems as well as by normal aging. Medications such as tranquilizers, sleeping pills, antidepressants, and even some over-the-counter drugs can affect balance, too.

Balance may be an issue if:
- You can't stand on one foot with your eyes closed for at least 5 seconds if you're 65 years old; 8 seconds if you're 55; and 12 seconds if you're 45. (Do this test next to a wall or with a partner close at hand to time you and make sure you don't fall.)
- You stop walking when you talk. The cognitive demands of doing both may be too taxing for your brain.

- Rough, uneven surfaces or stairs seem more daunting than you remember.
- You have already fallen—especially if you fell without knowing why.
- You have experienced brief spells of dizziness, light-headedness, blurred vision, or the feeling that the room is spinning.
- At times you feel disoriented, and may even forget where you are or what time it is.
- You feel as though you're moving when you're actually sitting or standing still.

MUSCULAR STRENGTH

One of my recommendations throughout this book is to forget about body-building and focus on functional fitness instead. I've also discussed why it's a mistake to be ego-driven and try to prove something by "lifting heavy." (Yes, guys, I'm talking to you.)

But that doesn't mean muscle-building exercise isn't necessary. In fact, it becomes even more important once you hit 50 or so. Many people don't realize that "use it or lose it" is literally what happens to our muscles. *Sarcopenia* is the term for age-related muscle loss, and researchers say it kicks in as early as the mid-twenties *if* we are not doing something to reverse the decline. It is estimated that by the time we're 50, 10 percent of our muscle mass is gone. From then on, the process accelerates and we lose another 15 percent every decade. If you've ever had a broken limb in a cast, you know how quickly muscles can atrophy when unused. That's just a sped-up and more dramatic version of what happens as you age.

Think about what life is like when you've lost half your muscle power—or maybe you already know. It takes some strength to do even simple things like lifting a bag of groceries, walking around the block, or getting in and out of a car, let alone household chores like cleaning or gardening. A healthy heart and lungs won't get you up a flight of stairs if your legs aren't strong enough to push your body weight counter to gravity. Muscular strength is also vital if you want to keep from falling. You can't stay upright and maintain your balance if you don't have enough muscle to support your joints and bones.

STRENGTH TRAINING BECOMES EVEN MORE IMPORTANT ONCE YOU'RE OVER 50.

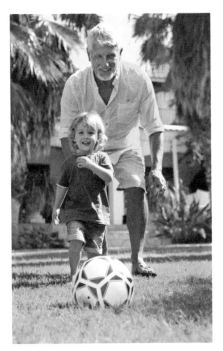

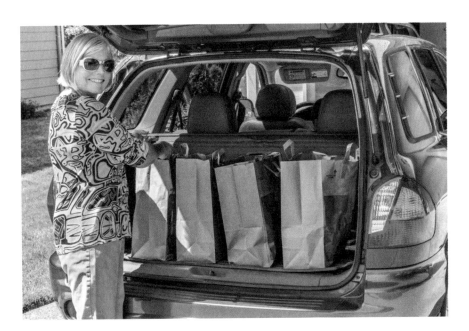

YOU CAN SUBSTANTIALLY INCREASE MUSCLE MASS AND QUALITY IN AS FEW AS 8 TO 12 WEEKS.

This is why being thin doesn't equate with being fit. A certain amount of muscle mass and strength is necessary to be physically functional at all. Muscle quality matters, too—which means bigger isn't necessarily better. Someone with beefy arms and legs may have muscles that are big in circumference but low in density and marbled with fat.

"Lean muscle mass" is the key phrase, and if it drops below a certain point, you're at risk of becoming frail—a medical syndrome that typically worsens over time because its symptoms interact in a vicious cycle. They include some combination of weakness and fatigue, slow walking speed, low physical activity levels, and unintentional weight loss as well as loss of muscle mass. And while we usually think of frailty as a problem of the elderly, it can also afflict someone of middle age with a debilitating medical condition.

Although medical science has found that losing some muscle mass and function is inevitable with age, new research suggests that those losses may be substantially reduced among people who stay active. One recent study of older athletes found that those in their seventies and eighties maintained a surprising degree of strength and muscle mass relative to the athletes in their sixties and even those in their fifties. When it comes to muscle loss, inactivity

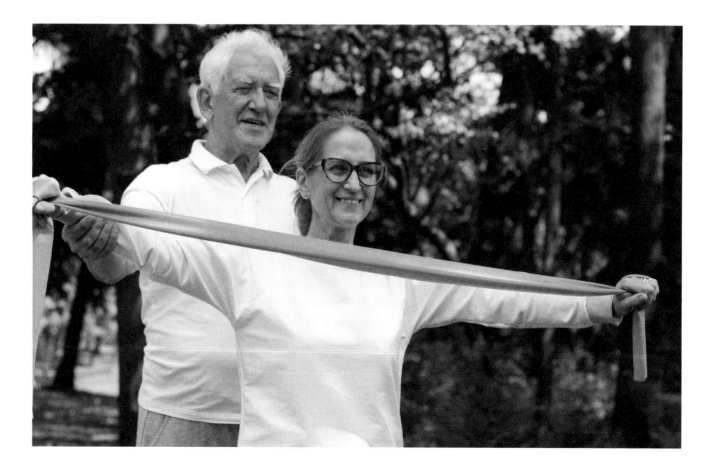

appears to be a bigger culprit than age. Scientists are still working to decipher the complex mechanisms behind muscle loss as they search for innovative treatments to slow or reverse the decline. What they do know, however, is that even for people in their sixties, seventies, and beyond, it's not too late to do something about it. Research shows that even in older adults, a moderately intense strength-training regimen can substantially increase muscle mass and quality in as few as 8 to 12 weeks. As I can attest, it will also give a big boost to your confidence and general feeling of well-being. Even people who start to exercise in their nineties can expect to see measurable improvements in physical function.

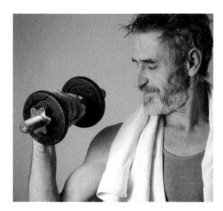

WHY MUSCULAR STRENGTH IS SO IMPORTANT

Preserve your independence. As important as cardiovascular exercise is to overall health, it's not enough to keep you from becoming weaker and losing physical function as you age. Muscle strength is critical if you want to keep up your lifestyle, avoid falls, and stay out of hospitals and nursing homes as you get older.

Help keep off excess pounds. Many people don't realize that muscles play a central role in metabolism. Think of your muscles as your body's power-house. Muscle cells burn the food calories you consume and deliver that energy to your body. Moreover, muscle tissue burns more calories than fat tissue, even when you're at rest. While the difference isn't huge—a pound of muscle burns about six calories a day while a pound of fat burns two—it adds up over time. So if you lose muscle and keep your caloric intake the same, it's only logical that you would increase your percentage of body fat and see your weight creep up over the years. You're also likely to expand around the middle since fat tissues are bulkier than muscle. Loss of muscle mass is one reason why the average person gains ten pounds per decade from age 25 onward. But let's look at the upside potential: while increasing muscle mass doesn't mean you can snack with impunity, it can certainly help you manage your weight.

Avoid or manage diabetes. Muscles are sensitive to insulin, so the more muscle mass you have, the better your body's response to the insulin in your system. Studies confirm that muscle-building exercise can help lower the risks of developing type 2 diabetes. It also increases the effectiveness of insulin taken by those who are already diabetic.

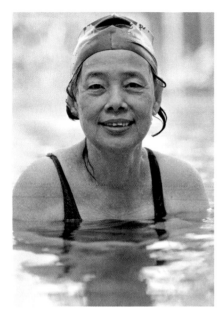

WE DON'T STOP
EXERCISING BECAUSE
WE GROW OLD.

WE GROW OLD
BECAUSE WE STOP
EXERCISING.

DR. KENNETH COOPER
The Cooper Institute

Support bones and joints. Low muscle mass tends to go along with low bone density and higher risks of falls and fractures, research shows. It also puts more stress on certain joints, such as the knees. Strength training and other weight-bearing forms of exercise are strongly advised for anyone who wants to avoid these problems—especially those at risk of developing *osteoporosis*, a disease that causes bones to become progressively thinner and more fragile. That risk is highest for women over 50, women or men with small body frames, and those with a family history of the disease. Cigarette smoking, alcohol abuse, and certain medications, such as steroids, can also increase osteoporosis risks.

WHAT TO DO FOR MUSCULAR STRENGTH

Train for strength three times a week. What we call strength training might more accurately be termed resistance training because the only way to build (or rebuild) your muscles is by causing them to contract against some source of external resistance. That means pushing, pulling, or lifting some kind of load, whether "free weights" (such as dumbbells or kettlebells), your own body weight, weight machines, exercise bands, or what have you. This works by tearing down muscle fibers so your body is stimulated to repair and grow muscle tissue, making it even stronger. Whatever you do, it's important to start with fairly light resistance and increase it gradually so you continue to challenge your muscles. While I'm a big proponent of exercises that use your own body weight, like good old-fashioned push-ups and planks, I also strongly believe that working out in a well-equipped, full-service gym with a knowledgeable trainer is the most effective way to do strength training. That said, any kind of resistance training that fits your lifestyle is worthwhile. Steps 3 and 4 in my program will tell you all about how to get started and make ongoing progress in strength training (see Chapters 7 and 8).

Keep moving. Gravity and the surfaces you walk on are sources of resistance, too! Conditioning activities like walking and cycling also contribute to muscle growth, as do household chores and active sports like tennis. Whatever you do, make sure you do it consistently. Studies show that muscle strength can decline measurably after two to six weeks of no exercise.

Get enough lean protein. Nutrition experts are increasingly urging older adults to get even more protein than the U.S. government's current adult guidelines recommend. Getting enough protein is especially vital for older people who are exercising and want to increase their lean muscle mass. Updated recommendations call for women to consume at least 70 grams of protein daily, while men should get 90 grams. What's more, scientists say it's important to eat protein at different times of the day. If you like to work out in the morning, make sure you don't skip the protein at breakfast. Protein-rich food sources include lean steak, chicken, and seafood (about 22 to 25 g. per 3 oz. serving). Other good sources are eggs (6 g. each) and high-protein dairy foods like cheese (8 g./oz.), cottage cheese (14 g. per half cup), and Greek yogurt (23 g./8 oz.).

What about vitamin D? Studies show that low vitamin D levels are also associated with low muscle strength. But be sure to talk with your doctor and get your levels tested before starting a vitamin D supplement—especially since too much vitamin D can be toxic to the body.

TEST YOUR STRENGTH   A = Excellent, B = Good, C = Needs work

This test measures lower body strength and, when performed with your arms crossed in front of you, balance. It's up to you and your comfort level whether you do this with or without your arms crossed.

Sit Down/Stand Up

To get started, just sit in a chair and stand up. Do this ten times.

A   I could stand up while keeping my arms crossed in front of me every time.

B   I was able to stand up without using my arms every time.

C   I always or almost always used my arms to push out of the chair.

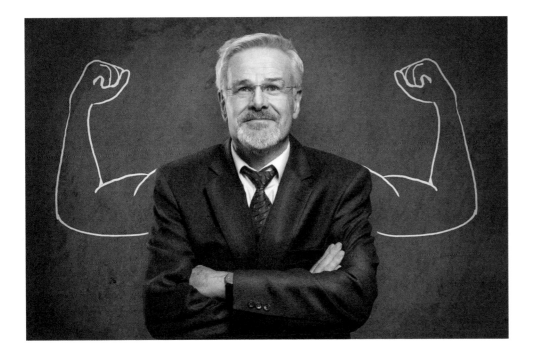

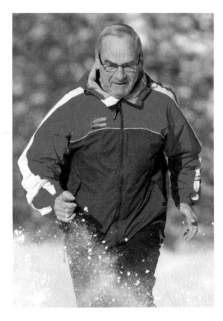

BE STRONG.
YOU NEVER
KNOW WHO YOU
ARE INSPIRING.

CARDIOVASCULAR ENDURANCE

Whether you call it "endurance," "conditioning," or "cardio," the idea is the same. To become or stay fit, you need to challenge your cardiovascular system, which powers everything else. You gain fitness the same way your body works: from the inside out.

Endurance activities include the types most of us associate with the word "exercise." They use large-muscle movements to raise your heart rate, accelerate your breathing, and cause you to work up a sweat.

What's often overlooked, however, is that there are two different kinds of endurance exercises that serve somewhat different purposes. If you truly want to become more fit, you need to understand what each of them entails and how you can benefit. *Aerobic* training is the kind most of us call "cardio." It aims to build cardiovascular endurance and efficiency by stepping up your heart rate and breathing for a period of 30 minutes or more. *Anaerobic* training is harder, more intense training that's done in short bursts. It, too, has some cardiovascular benefits, but it excels at building lean muscle mass and strength.

Many of the fitness guidelines I've seen put the focus on aerobic activity. But based on everything I've learned, working up to a program that includes both aerobic *and* anaerobic training is the way to get real results as long as your doctor has cleared you for vigorous activity. I say that for several reasons:

- Many people do aerobic activity that isn't very intense, like slow cardio on a treadmill or elliptical machine—and then wonder why they're not losing weight or gaining lean muscle. As virtuous as a long, slow slog on a cardio machine may feel, if you're not exercising hard enough to raise your heart rate significantly, there's not a whole lot of conditioning going on. Doing any kind of high-intensity, anaerobic exercises like fast jumping jacks or seal jacks is a way to make sure you're challenging your cardiovascular system while building lean muscle mass at the same time.

- Doing both kinds of exercises will give you more bang for the buck—that is, more results for the time you spend. The experts tell us that you get most of the cardiovascular benefits from the first 30 minutes of an aerobic workout. After that, you're in the realm of diminishing returns. Staying on

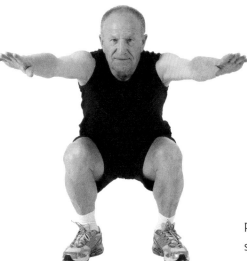

AEROBIC EXERCISE is any activity that revs up your heart rate and breathing and keeps them elevated for 30 minutes or more. That includes brisk walking, cardio machines like treadmills or ellipticals, jogging, swimming, cycling, rowing, climbing steps, aerobic dance classes—anything that keeps you moving at a moderately fast pace.

How it works "Aerobic" means "with oxygen." As your muscles work harder and pull oxygen from your blood, your breathing becomes faster and deeper, signaling your heart to pump more oxygen-rich blood into your arteries and to the tissues of your muscles and organs. As with other muscles, the more demands you place on your heart, the stronger and more efficient it becomes.

Benefits As the term "cardio" implies, aerobic exercise improves your cardiovascular health. It also burns calories. There has probably been more research on aerobic exercise than on any other aspect of fitness, and the many ways it benefits your body, brain, and mood are well documented.

ANAEROBIC TRAINING means high-intensity exercise done in short bursts of energy lasting anywhere from 20 seconds to a full minute or more. Examples include sprinting, star jumps, burpees, and squat jumps. You can incorporate brief intervals of anaerobic training into aerobic workouts, strength-building workouts, or both. Many cardio machines have built-in programs to do this.

How it works "Anaerobic" means "without oxygen." These activities demand oxygen beyond what your body can supply. As a by-product of anaerobic exercise, your muscles produce lactic acid, a waste substance that causes muscular fatigue and that feeling of muscle soreness you get after a hard workout.

Benefits Anaerobic exercises increase strength, lean muscle mass, and your body's ability to process and eliminate lactic acid. They improve cardiovascular fitness by increasing your body's maximum rate of oxygen consumption (VO_2 max). Because they're of short duration, they burn somewhat fewer calories than aerobic workouts. However, unlike aerobic exercise, anaerobic exercise has an "afterburner" effect so you burn more calories for 36 to 48 hours afterward, even while you're at rest. Anaerobic exercises are also especially good for building "fast twitch" muscle fibers—the ones that power more springy, explosive moves like those in a good tennis game.

WHAT MATTERS IS NOT
THE SHAPE YOU'RE IN,
BUT WHAT YOU CHOOSE
TO DO ABOUT IT.

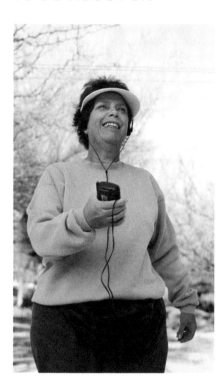

a cardio machine for 45 minutes or an hour may get you through a maga-zine or TV program. But if you really want to get fit, you'd be better off spending that extra time on higher-intensity conditioning that benefits you in different ways, or on flexibility exercises.

• Anaerobic exercises don't take long to do. What's more, they can easily be incorporated into a strength-training routine. Believe me, even 60 seconds of a high-intensity, whole-body exercise such as fast jumping jacks will keep your heart pumping hard well into the next segment of your workout.

That said, aerobic exercise is an essential component of any well-rounded fitness program. So how much of it should you be doing? According to the American College of Sports Medicine and the American Heart Association, adults over 65 (and those over 50 with chronic health issues) should get at least 30 minutes of aerobic activity three to five days a week—three if the activity is vigorous (such as jogging, fast walking, or aerobic dancing), and five if it is more moderate. By the way, it's fine to break your 30 minutes of aerobic exercise into smaller chunks, as long as your heart rate is continu-ously elevated for at least ten minutes at a time.

Let's not forget, however, that cardiovascular exercise is only one component of a well-rounded fitness program. You need time in your week to train for strength, flexibility, and balance, too. Thus, my program calls for working up to half an hour of brisk walking (or some similar aerobic exercise) three days a week. I also train for flexibility and balance on the days I walk and do strength training on the other days, keeping within my targeted time commitment of an hour a day, six days a week.

Remember, too, that vigorous strength workouts can also pump up your heart rate and breathing. For added conditioning I also incorporate a couple of high-intensity, anaerobic exercises into each of my three weekly strength workouts. It took me a year or more of strength training to work up to this, and I would advise anyone to get comfortable with a full-body workout before adding these more demanding moves. But I can tell you that once I did, my overall strength and endurance took a real leap forward, and kept progressing more rapidly than before. It was a difference I could see and feel!

One issue with aerobic exercise is keeping yourself honest. You need to consider whether your level of activity is intense enough to challenge your cardiovascular system. Monitoring heartbeats per minute is one traditional way to measure exertion, and there are now plenty of wearable heart-rate devices and smartphone apps, although their accuracy isn't assured.

However, even trainers often overlook the fact that heart rate is *not* recommended as a gauge of exercise intensity for older adults. For one thing, many older people are on prescription drugs that affect the cardiovascular system and skew calculations of the heart rate they should target during exercise. Beyond that, medical experts generally want to avoid quantitative measures that might lead older adults to overexert themselves. They believe that *perceived exertion* is a much better and safer yardstick for exercise intensity.

The American College of Sports Medicine and the American Heart Association guidelines for older adults measure exertion on a 0 to 10 scale, with 0 equal to sitting still and 10 being the maximum. "Moderate-intensity" exercise registers as a 5 or 6, producing "noticeable" increases in heart rate and breathing, while "vigorous intensity" is a 7 or 8, with more accelerated heart rate and respiration. Here, too, common sense can be your guide. If your workout feels "easy" and you can carry on a conversation while you move, step up the pace. If it feels like you're straining, quickly getting exhausted, or running out of breath, ease off a bit. The sweet spot is an intensity level that you can maintain for 30 minutes but that still feels challenging.

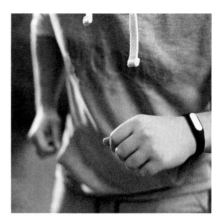

WHEN YOU FEEL
LIKE GIVING UP,
THINK ABOUT
WHY YOU STARTED.

WHY ENDURANCE IS SO IMPORTANT

A key to good health. While I strongly believe that aerobic exercise alone won't make you fit, I do agree with the experts who say it's an essential element of fitness. As discussed in Chapter 1, it can lower the risks of serious diseases, including heart disease, cancer, and diabetes. It has been shown to increase blood flow, lower blood pressure, reduce cholesterol levels, and boost immune function. Cardiovascular exercise is also good for your brain! Beyond improving brain function and lifting mood, it has been shown to help counter anxiety and depression. If these health benefits aren't compelling enough, think about what it would be like to look younger, feel more energetic, and have a better sex life, too.

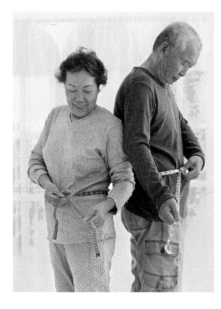

Controlling your weight. Aerobic exercise burns calories and is an important part of an overall weight-loss strategy. However, it may not burn as many calories as you think. For example, walking at a brisk pace of 3.5 miles per hour burns somewhere between 224 and 354 calories, depending on how much you weigh. That means you'd have to walk somewhere between 52 and 83 minutes just to burn off the 310 calories in one glazed jelly donut. To lose one pound, which equates to 3,500 calories, you'd have to walk rapidly for something like 10 to 15 hours. And don't forget that cardio activity can also increase your appetite! Exercise won't help you lose weight if you follow it with an extra snack or a supersize portion at mealtime. This is why the Mayo Clinic advises that "diet has a stronger effect on weight loss than physical activity does." At the same time, studies show that being physically active is essential to keeping off any pounds you lose. The upshot is that you need to watch what you eat *and* do aerobic exercise if you want to lose or keep off excess pounds.

WHAT TO DO FOR ENDURANCE

Start slow. It takes time to reverse years of inactivity, and if you are overly ambitious at the start, your good intentions will likely falter. Start with 10 or 15 minutes of walking three or four times a week and go from there. The important thing is that you get off the couch and ***do something.***

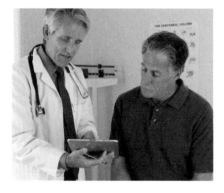

Have a simple plan, and reinforce it. Chapters 2 and 6 are full of strategies for making fitness a habit. One of the best ways is to make it fun by involving friends and giving yourself rewards. Organization helps, too. Put your weekly exercise sessions on your calendar and treat them as you would any other important appointment. In other words, make exercise a priority.

When to talk with your doctor. Unless you have chronic health issues or have been exceptionally inactive, you shouldn't need a doctor's okay to start a program of low- or moderate-intensity walking. But if you have any serious health concerns, it makes sense to check in with your doctor before beginning an exercise program, especially one that involves vigorous movement. Be especially cautious if you have any cardiovascular risk factors such as high blood pressure, any incidence of chest pain or irregular heartbeat, high cholesterol, high levels of LDL (the "bad" cholesterol), low levels of HDL (the "good" cholesterol), diabetes or a prediabetic condition, a past or current smoking habit, or a history of heart disease in your family. Your doctor may want to give you a stress test if you have any of these risk factors.

You should also ask your doctor whether any other conditions you may have, or any prescription medications you are taking, might affect your ability to exercise.

Keep raising the bar on your cardio. As your heart gets stronger and more efficient, your resting heart rate will drop. While your target heart rate won't change, it will take more effort to get to that targeted zone. That means you will need to increase the intensity of your aerobic exercise in order to keep challenging your cardiovascular system.

Add anaerobic exercises over time. While I don't believe it makes sense to pay a trainer to watch you while you're doing aerobic exercise, like riding a stationary bike or walking on a treadmill, a trainer can be a big help when it comes to high-intensity anaerobic exercise (think burpees). I've found it invaluable to have a coach and cheerleader who pushes me past my comfort zone and encourages me to try exercises I would never do on my own.

CLEAR YOUR MIND OF "CAN'T."

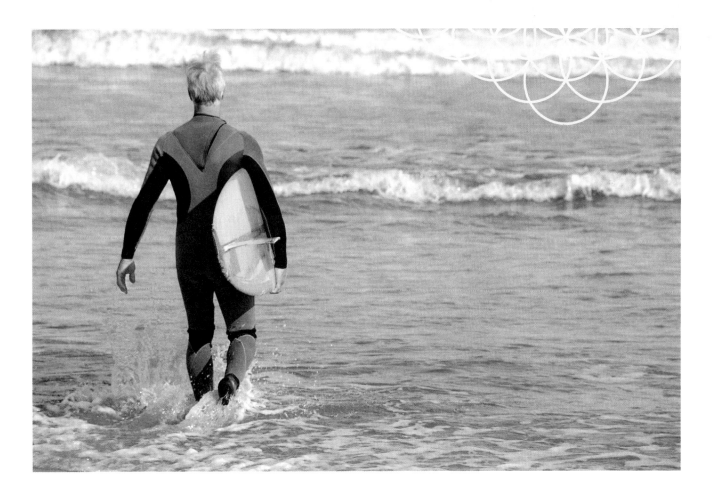

HOW GETTING FIT IS *DIFFERENT*

1

You finally have more time to devote.

That's good, because it takes an hour a day if you want to cover the basics.

2

There's no shortage of motivation.

Lowering the risks of life-threatening diseases isn't enough? How about easing those nagging aches and pains?

3

It's about how your body works, not how it looks.

You can (and should) leave the heavy lifting to the youngsters.

4

If you rest, you rust.

When you've got decades of wear and tear to offset, you've got to keep moving.

5

No one kind of exercise will do it all.

The cardio machine alone won't cut it. Strength, flexibility, and balance erode as you age if you're not actively training for each of them.

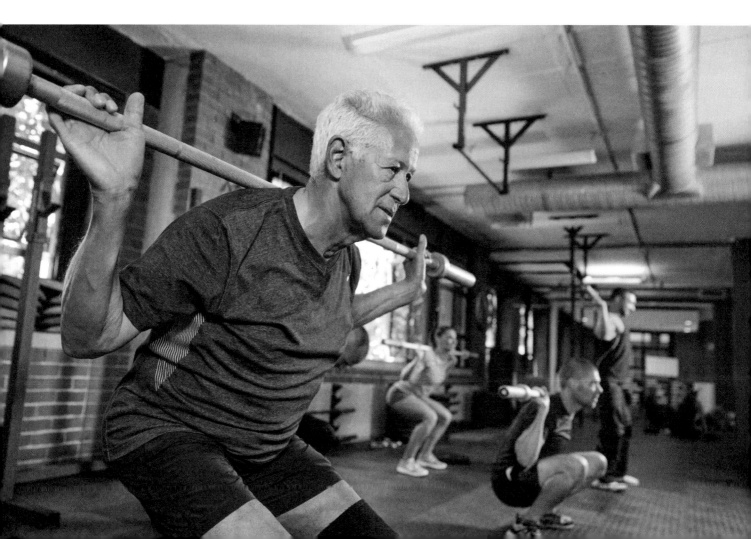

WHEN YOU'RE *OLDER*

6
Building lean muscle becomes even more important.
Otherwise, your strength and muscle mass steadily decline, your metabolism slows, and your waistline balloons.

7
It takes more understanding of body mechanics.
Older bodies are less forgiving. You need to know how to deal with weaknesses and avoid injuries.

8
Customizing your program is essential.
We each have our own needs and issues. What works for your spouse or friend might not work for you.

9
The stakes are higher.
How fit you are has a lot to do with the quality of your remaining years.

10
You're the one in charge.
Anything you do is better than nothing. You're the one in charge. What you want to accomplish and how hard you want to work are up to you.

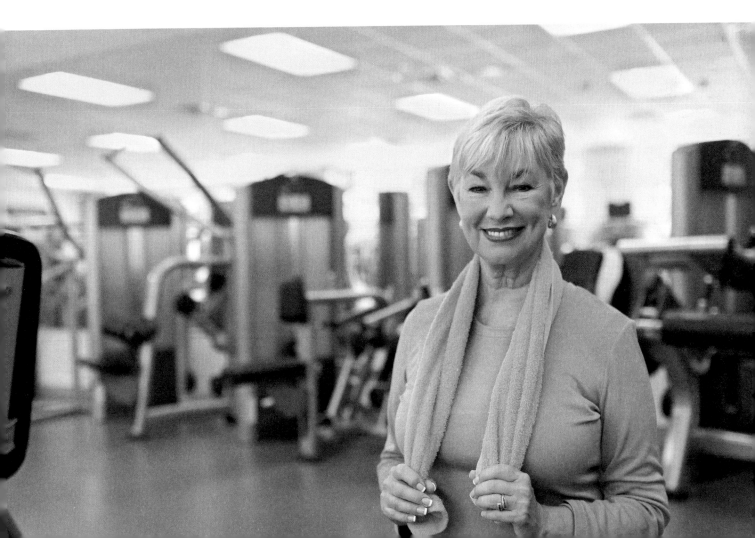

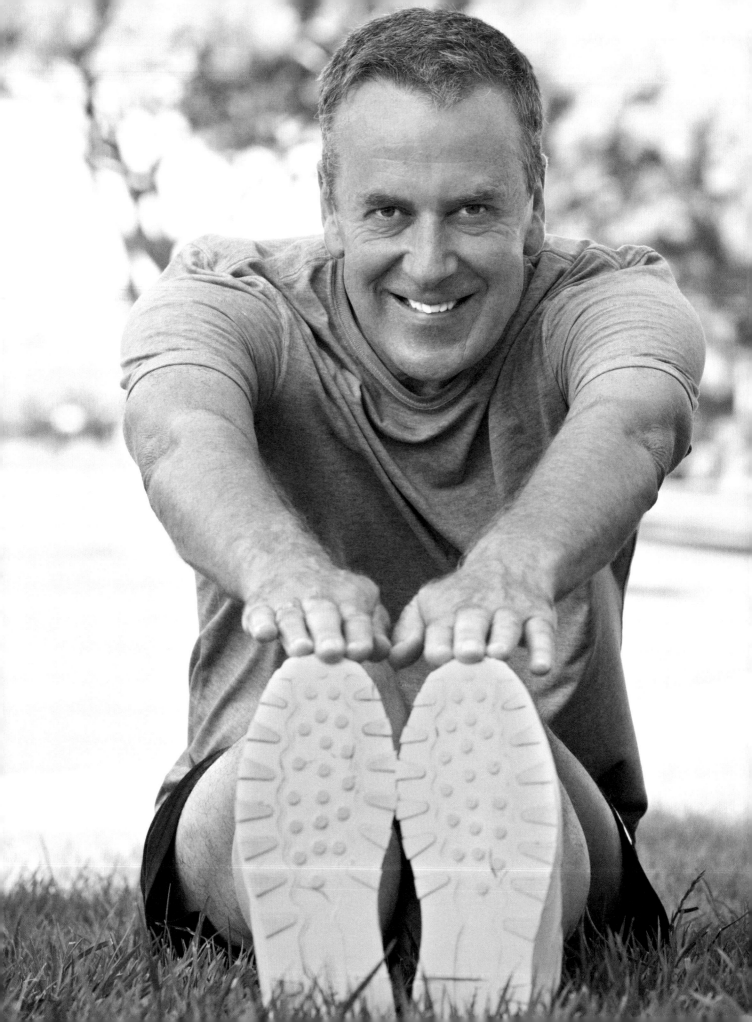

PART TWO

A FLEXIBLE, STEP-BY-STEP FITNESS PROGRAM

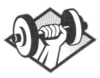

STEP 1   Tune In to Your Body

❖

STEP 2   Get In the Fitness Habit

❖

STEP 3   Begin Building Strength

❖

STEP 4   Advance to a Full-Body Workout

BELIEVE IN THE PERSON YOU WANT TO BECOME.

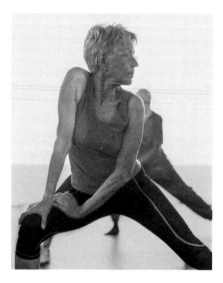

I HOPE Part One of this book has given you a fair share of the information—and, just as important, the inspiration—you need to make fitness a way of life. Part Two will show you how to accomplish that, one step at a time.

One of the reasons I felt compelled to write this book was the many hurdles I encountered in my own fitness quest. The biggest problem was the bewildering array of fitness advice out there—much more than I could absorb and interpret. I had no idea what to do, and no clear way to find out.

Determined to find my way through the chaos, I dove into it, and eventually arrived at some fundamental realizations.

We share many of the same physical problems as we age. By the time most of us reach midlife, our bodies have been reshaped and other habits acquired over many years. Postural and movement issues such as slumping shoulders, rounded backs, tight hip flexors, and knees that collapse inward are distressingly common. Many of us also suffer from age-related changes such as osteoarthritis and degeneration of spinal disks. But how bad these conditions get, and how their consequences are manifest, vary a great deal from person to person.

Idiosyncratic physical issues are another layer we have to deal with. First on the list are any structural problems you might have been born with, like having one leg that's shorter than the other. Other issues may arise over time; scoliosis, for example, is a curvature of the spine that usually occurs during the growth spurt just before puberty. On top of that are the physical traumas and injuries we sustain over the years—car accidents, fractures or sprains, lifting heavy furniture, you name it. Finally come personal habits like slouching or walking pigeon-toed, which may or may not have a structural cause.

No one fitness program is right for everyone. While some elements are essential to any complete fitness regimen, cookie-cutter solutions won't be effective if they don't happen to address your specific issues. It takes some time, exploration, and ongoing trial and error to figure out what exercise regimen works best for you. That's one reason why getting started is so hard. If you aren't sure what to do, and don't feel positive results from the things you try, you may soon abandon the effort.

There is no quick solution. The effects of sitting for hours a day for years on end can't be reversed overnight. Although you can feel the glow of increased blood flow and energy from even a single exercise session, it may take four to six weeks of regular, consistent exercise for you to start seeing real improvements in your physical functioning. Nor should anyone try to vault suddenly from a sedentary to an active way of life. That may do more harm than good, especially if you're at midlife or beyond. If you want to succeed at fitness, start with gradual changes in your activity level and add components as your body adapts. Then you've got to stick with it. Fitness can only come from the accumulation of many small gains over time. Slow and steady wins the race!

Exercise has to fit comfortably into your life. The best program in the world won't help you if it's not sustainable or demands more time than you're willing to give. To be effective, a program also has to fit your aspirations and personality. Some people thrive on challenge and want to see big measurable gains in their strength and range of motion; others just want to feel a little more spring in their step or keep the functionality they have.

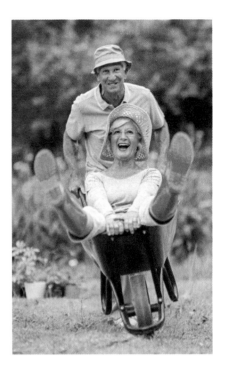

A PLACE TO START, A WAY TO PROGRESS

With all this in mind, I have designed a fitness framework that

- *Is flexible and adaptable, so it can be tailored to your needs*
- *Eases you into fitness one step at a time*
- *Guides you in making ongoing, cumulative fitness gains*
- *Addresses all five dimensions of functional fitness*
- *Requires just one hour a day, six days a week*

ONCE YOU START
EXERCISING ON
A REGULAR BASIS,
YOU WON'T WANT
TO GO BACK TO
YOUR OLD SELF.

The program this book lays out is the one I developed for myself some years back, and now follow religiously. Not being an expert in the mechanics of body movement, I can only share what I have learned and what has worked for me. But many people have issues similar to mine, and I've included guidelines and tips for adapting my program to your particular needs.

The program advances in four steps, each of which involves learning a relevant principle, practicing a specific type of movement, and incorporating a new activity or behavior into your life. The time commitment at the outset can be as little as 15 minutes a day, extending to one hour a day as you work through the program. The idea is to make fitness a way of life over a period of time rather than trying to learn or change everything at once.

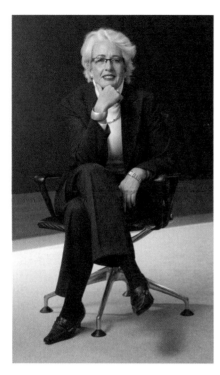

THINK OF YOUR
EXERCISE SESSIONS
AS "ME TIME."

YOU'RE THE BOSS

While the steps are designed to be additive, there is no law that says you have to work through all four. If you get through one or two steps and decide that's as far as you want or need to go, that's fine. Even if you only keep up those one or two routines, you will be better off than you were before. If, however, you follow my program through Steps 3 and 4, you should have the tools you need to stay fit and strong for life.

This framework is also designed so you can vary or personalize it at will. Once you have a complete fitness regimen, you can choose whether to go into maintenance mode, aiming to keep the functionality you have, or to keep working toward improvements. One of the rewards of my fitness journey has been discovering just how fascinating the kinetic aspects of the human body really are. You could spend a lifetime learning what is already known about fitness, and our knowledge base is expanding all the time.

And don't hesitate to think about augmenting this program with recreational sports or activities such as yoga, Pilates, dance, or tai chi, as long as you take care not to overuse muscles or put too much stress on joints. There's no law that says you can't substitute one activity for another. If bicycling is your thing rather than walking, that's fine, just so long as you keep moving.

Remember, too, that exercise sessions don't need to be marathons. Experts agree that 30 minutes of stretching or walking is enough to give you the benefits of those activities. It's fine to do more, but you will soon reach the point of diminishing returns. If you're ambitious and have the time to devote, you may be better off doing some other kind of physical activity.

So, where do you go from here? That comes down to a single question only you can answer.

Is it worth investing six hours a week to be able to move with ease, reduce or prevent aches and pains, and learn how to stay strong and flexible for life?

If your answer is yes, then you're ready to turn the page and embark on a journey of transformation.

Invest 1 Hour a Day, 6 Days a Week

The path, the pace, and the extracurriculars are all up to you

STEP 1 ~ *TUNE IN TO YOUR BODY*

PRINCIPLE ~ Make the Mind/Body Connection   **PRACTICE ~** Ease into Fitness with Stretching

START	PROGRESS	ONGOING	OPTIONAL
Stretch at least 10-15 minutes daily	Work up to a 30-minute routine at least 3x a week	Stretch 30 minutes on the 3 days a week that you walk	Pilates, yoga, tai chi, deep-tissue massage

STEP 2 ~ *GET IN THE FITNESS HABIT*

PRINCIPLE ~ Take Charge of Your Posture and Breathing   **PRACTICE ~** Make Walking a Priority

START	PROGRESS	ONGOING	OPTIONAL
Walk at least 10-15 minutes, 6 days a week	Work up to 30-minute walks, 6 days a week	Walk 30 minutes 3x per week on days you don't do strength training	Cardio machines, bicycling or spinning, hiking or jogging, stair climbing, any active sport

STEP 3 ~ *BEGIN BUILDING STRENGTH*

PRINCIPLE ~ Focus on Good Form Above All   **PRACTICE ~** Master a Few Classic Moves

START	PROGRESS	ONGOING	OPTIONAL
Practice 5 exercises 3x a week, modifying as needed	Work up to more challenging versions	Include these moves in your 3 weekly training sessions	TRX classes

STEP 4 ~ *ADVANCE TO A FULL-BODY WORKOUT*

PRINCIPLE ~ Find Multiple Ways to Progress   **PRACTICE ~** Make Sure Your Workout Covers the Bases

START	PROGRESS	ONGOING	OPTIONAL
One-hour sessions 3x a week	Target weaknesses and add challenge where you can	Keep advancing and varying your 3x weekly sessions	High-intensity interval training

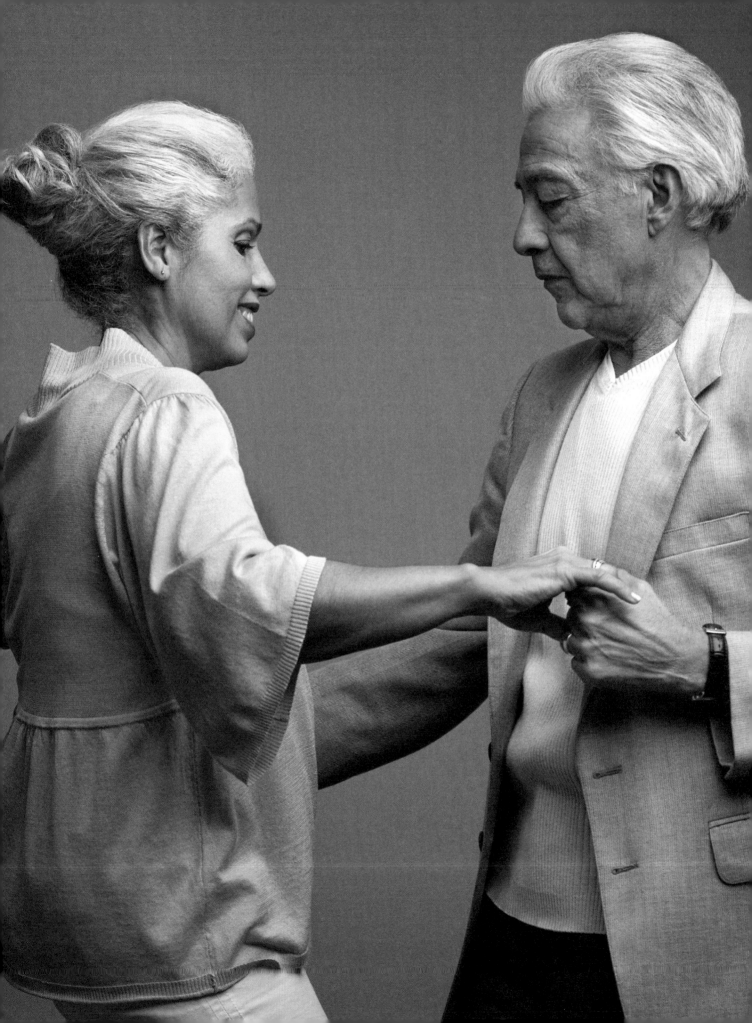

CHAPTER FIVE

Step 1
Tune In to Your Body

WHEN WAS THE LAST TIME you watched small children playing? You can see how they fully inhabit their bodies, moving for the sheer joy of it. Cavorting like puppies, they effortlessly run, climb, jump, and twist without ever giving their movements a thought.

Somewhere along the line, as our lives get busier and we become preoccupied with school, work, and other responsibilities, most of us lose that exhilarating sense of aliveness. The less we move, and the more time we spend commuting, working, or watching what's on a screen, the more disconnected we get from our bodies. We start treating them like conveyances that exist just to move our brains from place to place rather than as the sophisticated and marvelously capable machines they really are.

Then, when we do move, we go about it unconsciously. We simply do what comes naturally—and that's a big part of the problem. Years of a chair-bound, power-assisted way of life take their toll. Between too much sitting and too much stress, our bodies get progressively tighter and more prone to aches and pains. They begin to lose the connectedness and range of motion we need in order to move without stressing vulnerable joints. If we haven't made a habit of standing up straight, we gradually lose some of the muscular strength we need to do so. And too often we cope with these problems by trying to ignore them, distancing ourselves even further from our physical selves.

Moving more, and in a variety of ways, can do much to remedy the physical dysfunctions that come with age—but only if we are consciously engaged and aware as we move. Otherwise, it's just more of the same. Exercising mindlessly produces limited results because it reinforces our physical dysfunctions and poor movement habits rather than correcting them. At worst, it amplifies our weaknesses and puts us at risk for injuries. In the next two chapters you will learn why moving with precision and good form is so important—and you can't have good form if you're not moving deliberately and consciously.

IN THIS CHAPTER

- *Techniques for unifying mind and body with your breathing*

- *The role of the sensory feedback loop*

- *How to begin engaging and controlling your muscles*

- *Why stretching is integral to any fitness program*

- *What the kinetic chain has to do with our aches and pains*

Here's the other thing: exercise *is* boring, if you do it mindlessly. Slogging through a checklist of exercises while you check your email or glance up at the TV monitors turns exercise into something you just want to get done and over with, like cleaning out the garage or your clothes closet.

But when you are mentally focused and fully present in each movement, exercising is a completely different experience. Your mind and body are joined as you actively orchestrate how your body moves through space. It's a kind of ballet, very much like what you see in a championship tennis match or on a pro basketball court. It's also a time for active learning. Each moment, and each exercise, is another chance to throw off the weight of the years and train your body to move correctly, as it is designed to do. When you approach exercise with that mind-set, it's not just another chore. Every session is one more step toward becoming a better version of yourself.

This is why knowing how to be in touch with your body should be a foundational first step in any fitness program. My program starts there, and with the practice of daily stretching—a great way to learn more about your body and begin improving how you move.

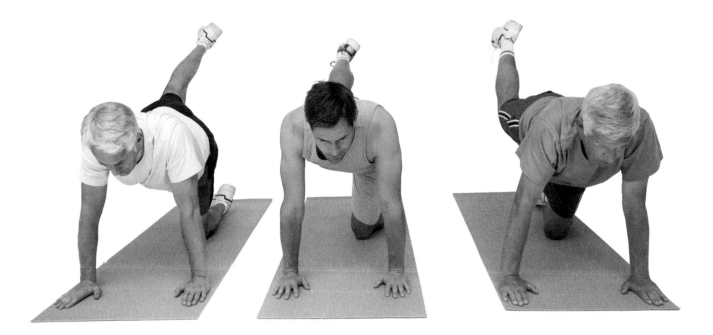

MAKE THE MIND/BODY CONNECTION

If you want to improve how your body moves and functions, you must first put your mind in charge. That's the only way you can achieve the body awareness it takes to override old habits and replace them with new, more functional patterns of movement.

But being body aware isn't only about getting better results from your exercise. It's about how you move through your life. Every physical action you take— whether standing up from a chair, getting in or out of a car, or lifting a bag of groceries—calls upon your body to coordinate a complex series of movements. The more consciously you move through your day, the sooner your body will learn new and better ways of moving. Over time, they will be embedded in your muscle memory and become part of who you are.

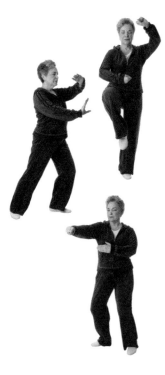

There's even more to this story. Increasing your body awareness is one of the keys to mindfulness—the ability to be focused on the present physical sensations. Medical practitioners are increasingly enlisting mindfulness-based techniques and therapies to help people reduce stress and anxiety, ease depression, alleviate insomnia, and treat stress-related medical conditions. The phrase *mens sana in corpore sano*, "a healthy mind in a healthy body," is ancient wisdom that goes back to the Greeks and Romans, yet couldn't be more relevant to our lives today.

So how can you forge and nurture the connection between mind and body? It takes a combination of mental focus and physical awareness. With some practice it's not hard to do, and the more you practice it, the easier and more natural it becomes. Here are some ways to get started:

BODY AWARENESS
ISN'T JUST
ABOUT EXERCISE.
IT'S HOW YOU MOVE
THROUGH LIFE.

PRACTICE CONSCIOUS BREATHING

Breathing is one major life process that we can regulate either automatically or with the conscious mind. When you center your conscious attention on your breathing, you call on your brain's higher cognitive centers, bringing your mind and body together by joining them in a common task. If you are able to sustain that focus for even a brief period of time, you can experience a state of calm awareness, as the background chatter that usually goes on in the mind is quieted or stops altogether.

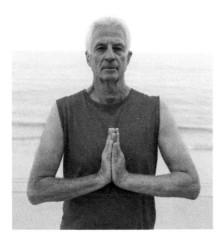

CONTROLLING YOUR
BREATHING IS ONE
OF THE KEYS TO
MINDFULNESS.

This is why breathing techniques have been part of meditation and spiritual practice for centuries. These days we also use them to help sharpen concentration, achieve deep relaxation, and more easily get to sleep at night.

Try the simple, but powerful breathing exercises on page 99. Not only will they help you be more in touch with your body, they also will give you a head start on the kind of breathing you will need for stretching, strength training, and good posture.

FEEL YOUR BODY IN ACTION

Body awareness is a critical ingredient in motor control, the complex process by which our brains interact with our sensory systems, the musculoskeletal system, and the world around us as we move. To get real results from any exercise you do, you must be able to activate different muscles and parts of your body with some degree of control and precision rather than just letting a movement happen. If at this point you're not sure how to respond to instructions like "engage your core" or "contract your gluteal muscles," stay with me; you'll soon know what they mean.

Motor control relies in part on what physiologists call a "sensory feedback loop." First your body's proprioceptive systems sense where you are in space (see "Balance" on pages 69–72). Your brain issues a command ("I want to…") and, through its neural networks, stimulates your nerves, muscles, and organs to act. As you move, you get feedback on how your body's position is changing, how much force your muscles need to exert, and how your heart and lungs are responding. All this can take place in the blink of an eye! When you exercise, you are training these systems as well as your muscles.

At this point we'll start by feeling and engaging every muscle in your body. This is a simplified version of a whole-body exercise called "salute to the sun," which yoga instructors often use as a warm-up for a session.

1   Stand with your feet pointed straight ahead, parallel and in line with your hips. Straighten up by lifting your chest and pulling your shoulders down and back; lift your chin, too, so your eyes are looking straight ahead. Slightly rotating your arms outward will help you get your shoulders in position; that may also happen automatically.

2 The next step is to engage the powerful muscles of your core, using the "pelvic tuck," a move that is subtle but important to learn because it puts your spine in a natural and neutral position. The easiest way to do this is to inhale, and then pull your bellybutton upward as you exhale. Did you feel your tailbone drop and the big gluteal muscles of your buttocks contract? They're not just for sitting! You should also feel your knees rotating outward and your leg muscles engaging all through your outer thighs, calves, and ankles. The pelvic tuck also lengthens your spine and neck, and even pulls up the arches of your feet! (Read more about this in the next chapter.)

3 Now keep your pelvis tucked and your core engaged as you lift your arms and hands straight into the air above your shoulders. Give them a slight stretch skyward as you slowly inhale and exhale.

4 For the final stage in this sequence, move your arms down into a Y, as you would when doing a jumping jack. Rotate your arms outward and look upward as you tilt your head back slightly. Your upper back will also arch slightly, but don't overdo it, especially at first.

Notice that this exercise also moves your body upward and outward, reversing the inward-and-downward pull of habit and gravity. As you repeat this move, you can practice further flexing the muscles of your shoulders, core, and legs. True to its name, the sun salute is one of the best ways to start your day.

CHECK IN WITH YOUR BODY THROUGHOUT THE DAY

Like any other habit, body awareness grows as it is practiced and reinforced. I'm not talking about being obsessive. Body awareness simply means paying attention to your body and having some gratitude for what it can do. It also means noticing opportunities to help your body feel and function better.

Are you moving with intent and control? Can you rely more on your core muscles, and less on your arms, when you stand up or sit down? Do you need a snack or a meal to boost your energy?

If your body is feeling tight, you can take it as a signal to stop, breathe, and stretch so that tension is released. If you're feeling tired and achy, a few minutes of stretching or a brisk walk might make all the difference. Or maybe your body is telling you to slow down and give yourself a rest.

The more you start thinking of your body as this wonderful machine that you own and live in each day, the better you can become at its care and feeding. As you start to feel the benefits, that sense of wonder and gratitude will more frequently light up your day. The experiences and sensations of daily life can hold many rewards, like a movie that keeps bringing new scenes for you to savor. All you have to do is pay attention.

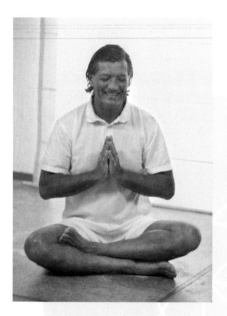

YOGA SET ME FREE

I always knew that long hours at a desk and frequent business trips were hard on the body, but that's what my law practice demanded. Add to that the pressures of life and everything going on in the world. The stress started to feel like steel bands constricting my back, neck, and shoulders.

Like a lot of guys, I guess, I'd never really thought about trying yoga. What finally convinced me was seeing an older man back his car out of a parking space. His neck was so tight, he had to turn his whole body to look behind him. I didn't want to be that guy!

So I went off to my first yoga class, and I was shocked to discover just how stiff and tight I was, especially my hips. Many poses I could barely do, or not at all.

Now I'm a very different person, and it's a direct result of my weekly yoga classes and daily sessions at home. Physically, I'm way more flexible. My balance has improved, and I'm much more conscious of how I'm moving.

Then there's the spiritual piece. I used to get upset and depressed when things went wrong or the news was bleak. Yoga and meditation taught me a different way to be in the world. I'm still aware of what's happening out there, but I know I don't have to own it. Things no longer have the same emotional charge for me. Once I learned how to connect mind, body, and spirit, everything in my life got better.

RICHARD, 54

TRY THESE EXERCISES one at a time over a period of days, getting comfortable with each one before you move on to the next. Even a minute or two of practice will help. You should soon be able to work up to sessions of five minutes or more. If you have a hard time corralling your attention at first, don't worry. Just notice what happens without attaching any judgment to it, and try again. You can practice at any point during the day, whenever you've got a quiet moment or can take time out from another activity. This is especially helpful if you are feeling stressed. While your thoughts can cause muscles to tense, you can also harness them to help you release tension and relax.

Many people find it helpful to have an audio guide that leads them through the steps in conscious breathing. Any number of CDs or free MP3s are available on the Internet. A yoga or meditation class is another good way to learn these techniques.

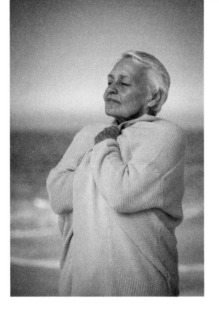

1   Sit or lie down in a comfortable position, in a quiet place with no distractions. If your shoulders are pulled up or tensed, let them drop. Now breathe through your nose as you naturally do, and bring your attention to the physical act of breathing. Don't try to do anything about your breathing; just spend two or three minutes feeling each in-breath and out-breath. You can close your eyes to help you focus.

2   Now try the same thing, but mentally follow each cycle of in- and out-breaths from beginning to end. It doesn't matter if your breaths are short or long, deep or shallow. Just try to stay with them so your mind and your breath are linked. If your attention wanders, don't worry. Just gently call it back. As you concentrate on your breathing, it will naturally become deeper and slower.

3   The next step is to extend your awareness to your body as you breathe. As you inhale and exhale, feel your body as fully alive. Notice your heart beating, as it pumps oxygen-rich blood and healing energy to every part of your body. Mentally do a quick body scan, from the top of your head to the tips of your toes. If you sense areas of tightness, mentally release that tension as you exhale. Just as your thoughts can make your muscles tense up, your conscious attention can also make them relax. This is something you can practice at work, at home, or whenever you need it.

4   Now try controlling your breathing. Breathe in slowly and deeply through your nose. Try to fill your lungs as fully as you can, letting your chest lift as you do. Hold your breath to the count of three. Then exhale slowly through lips slightly pursed, as if you were about to whistle, relaxing the muscles in your face, jaw, and shoulders as you exhale. The ability to control your breath comes into play whenever you do stretching or strength training.

IF YOU'RE NOT
BOTHERED BY
ACHES AND PAINS
BY THE TIME YOU'RE
45 OR 50, JUST
WAIT UNTIL YOU'RE
60 OR 70!

EASE INTO FITNESS WITH STRETCHING

You might be surprised that I recommend stretching as the first step in your fitness journey. That's because I have learned firsthand just how powerfully therapeutic it can be. Stretching is an easy, gentle form of exercise you can do anywhere. Yet it's one of the best things you can do for your body because it elongates muscles, helps tendons stay elastic, and increases the range of motion at the joints. It also eases the tightness that can distort your movements, sometimes triggering a painful cascade of consequences. For people like me a stretching regimen can be life-changing, and that is no exaggeration.

I'm not alone in these views. Fitness experts agree that anyone who is generally inactive absolutely needs to stretch. Bad backs, aching knees, painfully tight necks and shoulders, sciatica—so many of our everyday ailments trace back to too much sitting and too much stress. If you're not bothered by aches and pains by the time you're age 45 or 50, just wait until you're 60 or 70! Staying flexible is also essential if you want to preserve your mobility while avoiding injuries and falls (see Chapter 4).

People who are active also need to stretch, kinesiologists say, and that goes double for amateur or professional athletes. It's not just that being limber helps athletes perform better, because their movements are less restricted.

SINGLE-LEG BRIDGE

HAPPY BABY (top)
KNEE TO CHEST

FLOOR COBRA

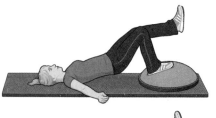

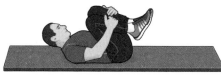

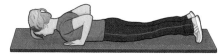

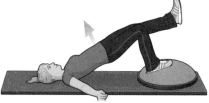

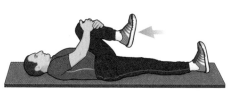

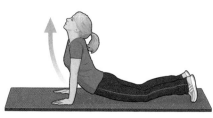

They also need stretching to counteract the effects of pounding, repetitive movements and soft tissue injuries. Once muscles or tendons have been sprained or strained, scar tissue prevents them from regaining full flexibility. So if you've ever had this kind of injury to an ankle, knee, wrist, or some other joint, stretching is even more important.

Then there's the third category of people—those who suffer from chronic pain due to some trauma, like "throwing out" your back in an ill-advised move. That was me, all right. Several incidents over the years had caused episodes of severe and lingering back pain. The last time it happened was seven years ago, a point when I was still ignorant about the correct ways to move and lift. Trying to move a piece of furniture was all it took to leave me with bouts of pain so agonizing that I literally had to crawl to the bathroom at times. One wrong move disrupted my life for months.

In my case, stretching turned out to be a big piece of the answer. Not only does it feel great to be looser and more flexible, but also my back pain has virtually disappeared. Now it is unthinkable for me not to do my full 30-minute stretching routine three times a week, augmented by a weekly movement class. But, as the research tells us, stretching is integral to anyone's fitness strategy, whether you suffer from chronic, trauma-induced pain or simply want to minimize the garden-variety aches and stiffness that come with age.

This is not to say that stretching is a quick and easy fix; it took me six weeks to see a meaningful change, and there are right ways and wrong ways to do it (see "Stretching Dos and Don'ts" on page 104). You also have to figure out what your body really needs and which stretches work best for you. I hope I can help you streamline that process by sharing what I've learned along the way.

STRETCHING IS INTEGRAL TO ANY FITNESS STRATEGY.

CAT / COW POSE

LOWER BACK STRETCH
CHILD'S POSE

SEATED HIP STRETCH

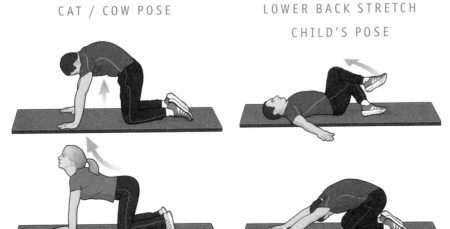

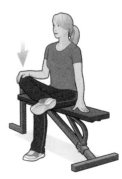

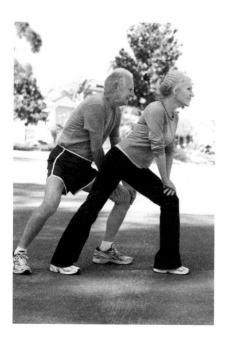

Rule out medical causes first. If you're experiencing severe or chronic pain, the cause might be a medical problem, like osteoarthritis, or a structural problem, like one leg shorter than the other. If you've recently had surgery, ask your surgeon if you should avoid or limit stretching. If you have an ongoing health condition, it's always a good idea to check with your doctor before embarking on a fitness program.

Look for root causes. Beyond looking at symptoms, you'll need to figure out what might be behind them. Fitness trainers usually kick off a first session by asking what goals you want to accomplish. But if you're past 50, it makes much more sense to start with your issues so you can get to their root cause. Realize, however, that this may take some time and some detective work. Once you understand the kinetic chain (see page 105), you will know why. For years I had no idea my bad back stemmed almost entirely from lower-body tightness that threw my spine out of alignment. Neither did any of the medical specialists I consulted about my pain; they were experts in conditions like spinal stenosis and degenerative disk disease, not flexibility issues. Not until my trainer watched me exercise over several months did the ultimate problem come to light.

Consult movement experts. If your problems are severe, I'd recommend seeing a good physical therapist; even one or two sessions may be immensely helpful. Stretching is also a good way to start working with a trainer. A knowledgeable trainer can help you diagnose problems, develop a routine, and make sure you're doing it correctly. While I do most of my stretching on my own, I ask my trainer to help fine-tune my routine every three months or so.

Ease into it. I recommend starting with sessions of 10 to 15 minutes daily, covering all major muscle groups. That seems about right for most people. If you experience severe pain or tightness, you might want to stretch for 30 minutes as I typically do. In any case, give yourself some time to work up to a full routine. As you feel the results, you'll want to do more.

HIP FLEXOR

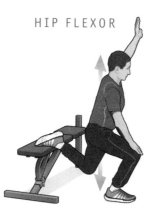

DOWNWARD-FACING DOG

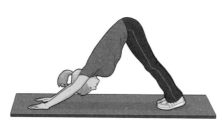

ABDUCTOR STRETCH

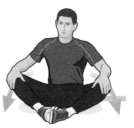

Mix stretches. The stretches in this chapter include both static and dynamic stretches. Static stretches are the more familiar kind; they involve achieving and holding a position that stretches a muscle or muscle group. There are two kinds of static stretches: active, in which the muscle being stretched does the work of holding the position, and passive, which are assisted by someone else or some other external force, like a strap, elastic band, barre, or gravity. Dynamic stretches involve moving muscles and joints from one position to another, through a full range of motion; an example is the lunge (see page 161). Stretches of this type are useful in helping you warm up and loosen muscles before walking, working out, or activities like golf or tennis. Be sure to incorporate both types.

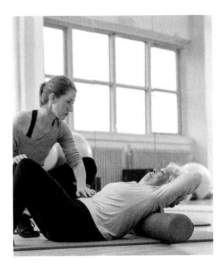

Expect your routine to evolve over time. As you try various stretches, you'll learn which ones work best for you. Several of the stretches shown in these pages are straight out of the yoga and Pilates classes I've taken. And some of my favorites are ones I've come up with on my own, just by trying different movements to ease the areas of tightness I'm feeling. Any stretch that helps you feel looser and more flexible is worth incorporating into your repertoire. Remember, the best stretches are the ones you like and will do consistently.

Keep it up. Don't fail to stretch, even if circumstances force you to skip your walk or workout. Studies show that six weeks of regular stretching can make a big difference in your flexibility, but you'll quickly revert to where you were before if you let your routine lapse.

A LACK OF FLEXIBILITY MAY BE THE HIDDEN CAUSE OF PAIN OR INJURIES.

Control your breathing. The basic rules for stretching are similar to those for strength training: inhale as you are poised for a stretch, exhale as you move, and don't hold your breath. Keep breathing naturally as you extend and hold a stretch. Breathing in a slow, measured way will help you move into a stretch and comfortably stay with it as long as you want to hold it.

CALF STRETCH

HIP STRETCH

WALL STRETCH

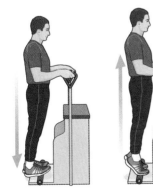
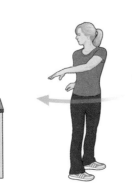
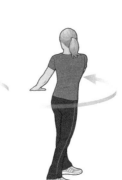
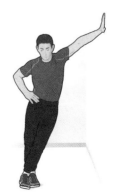

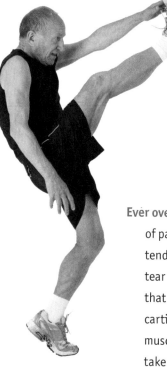

DO

Stretch slowly and gently until your muscles feel tight but not painful.

Hold your stretch for 20 to 30 seconds at the farthest point.

Stretch at least 15 to 20 minutes three times a week, ideally working up to sessions of 30 minutes.

Pay attention to good posture and form (see Chapters 6 and 7 for more on this).

Think about the order in which you do your stretches. I find it helpful to start with the stretches that engage and extend your core muscles, close to the center of your body, and then move outward to shoulders and limbs.

Stretch those muscles that feel tight after a workout or playing sports, like tennis or golf. A few brief stretches can help minimize soreness and stiffness the next day.

Find opportunities for mindful stretching in your daily activities (like reaching for something on a shelf) and as you warm up for other types of exercise (like walking and resistance training).

DON'T

Ever overextend or stretch to the point of pain, which can injure muscles and tendons. Overextension can also sprain or tear ligaments, the tough bands of tissue that connect bones to other bones or cartilage. Ligaments are less elastic than muscles or tendons; when injured, they can take weeks or months to heal.

Bounce or jerk. Once you've stretched as far as you comfortably can, it's okay to back off slightly and then extend again if you do it slowly and mindfully.

Strain or "cheat" to reach the end point of a move. A classic example is bending your knees as you try to touch your toes. The goal isn't to reach your toes; it's to elongate your muscles. You'll get better results if you don't take shortcuts.

Assume that having arthritis is a reason not to stretch. While those suffering from the disease may need to limit the range of motion in certain movements, stretching can help lessen the pain and stiffness. Ask your doctor or physical therapist to suggest stretches you can do safely.

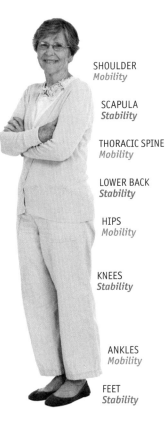

SHOULDER
Mobility

SCAPULA
Stability

THORACIC SPINE
Mobility

LOWER BACK
Stability

HIPS
Mobility

KNEES
Stability

ANKLES
Mobility

FEET
Stability

WHAT'S BEHIND THOSE ACHES AND PAINS? One of my biggest "aha" moments was discovering that the real cause of my bad back is the extreme tightness of my hips rather than some spinal problem. How could that be, when these two body parts seem totally unrelated? At first it made no sense to me. But then I learned about the kinetic chain—the way that all parts of the body, including muscles, joints, nerves, and connective tissues, work together to produce a movement.

To understand how this works, it helps to think of the body as a series of overlapping segments that are linked at the joints. Some areas are designed for stability, while others provide mobility. This is why the human body can perform such complex movements. All of its components are connected, and each one supports the others. But a chain is only as strong as its weakest link. If one part of your body's kinetic chain is weak or not functioning correctly, the next link in the chain must compensate. And then you're on the road to physical imbalances, pain, and injury.

The hips, for example, are a prime trouble spot for many people, including professional athletes, because years of sitting have left so many of us with tightness in the pelvic area. Can you trace a figure eight or a circle in the air with your hips? I certainly couldn't. And if you don't have mobility in your hips, your spine has to move instead, forcing it into unnatural and often damaging positions.

This is why physical therapists and trainers will warn you to bend from the hips, where your body is naturally hinged, and never from the waist. It's also one more reason not to do sit-ups, which press your lower back against the floor rather than maintaining its natural lumbar curve (see Chapter 7).

There's much more to learn about the kinetic chain, such as the difference between open- and closed-chain movements. But for someone just getting into fitness, the key takeaway is that all parts of your body are connected. If you want to get to the underlying cause of aches and pains, you need sound advice from someone who understands body mechanics and can look at your issues holistically.

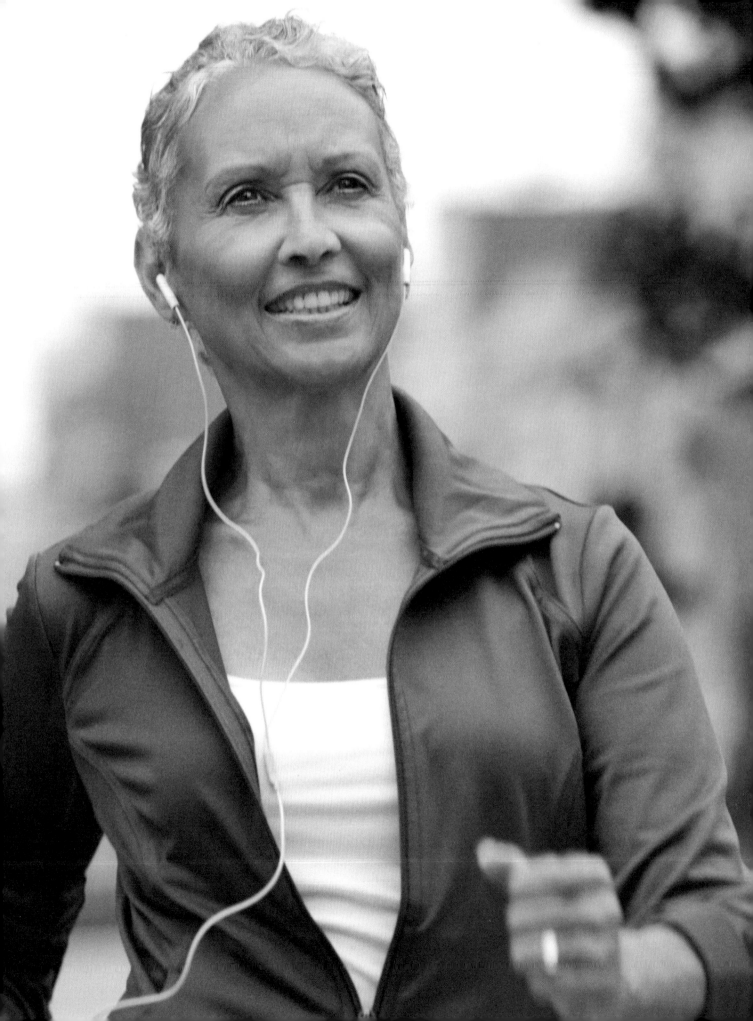

CHAPTER SIX

Step 2
Get In the Fitness Habit

ONE OF THE BIG REASONS people launch into fitness programs and then end up abandoning them is trying to do too much all at once. New habits aren't created overnight. It's a step-by-step process you have to stick with, evolve, and reinforce over time. Another common mistake is plunging into an ambitious set of exercises without knowing how to do them correctly or even why you're doing them. Understanding some of the basics behind good body mechanics will set you up for success.

This chapter aims to ease you into fitness as a way of life. As the way in, we'll start by learning how to improve the things we all do every day: standing, sitting, and breathing. That's not as elementary as it sounds; it actually takes some time, some knowledge, and a good deal of focus. You may be surprised how big a difference good posture and breathing can make in your life.

Then we'll move on to a walking program—working up to 30 minutes a day, six days a week. Once you've established that habit, you'll be solidly on the fitness path.

IN THIS CHAPTER

- *Why posture and breathing are key building blocks of fitness*

- *Right and wrong ways to stand, sit, and breathe*

- *Ways to assess your own posture against the ideal*

- *How conscious breathing can help you improve your physical and mental functioning*

- *Tips for starting and keeping up a walking regimen*

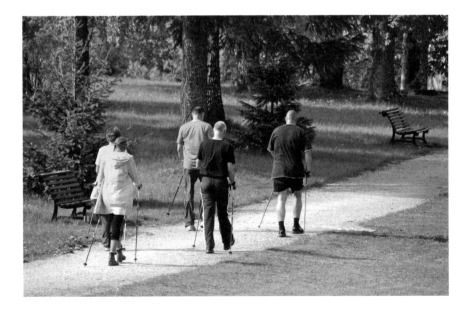

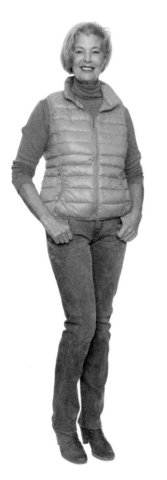

HOW YOU CARRY
YOURSELF CAN HAVE
A PROFOUND EFFECT
ON HOW YOU LOOK
AND FEEL.

PRINCIPLE

TAKE CHARGE OF YOUR POSTURE AND BREATHING

Straight and tall—that's the way to move through life, as generations of mothers and drill sergeants have exhorted us.

It's not a matter of being morally upright. The fact is, weak, slumping posture is hard on the body—much harder than many of us realize. It pulls you downward and inward, throwing your physique out of alignment. Then your body weight and the forces of movement are unevenly distributed, making it more difficult to move while putting stress on your back, muscles, joints, and internal organs. Poor posture is a leading cause of pain and fatigue. It can even compromise your breathing and digestion over time. How well would your car function with a bent axle, an underinflated tire, and a cracked motor mount? Structural integrity and stability are no less important to your body.

In simplest terms, good posture means standing up straight with your hips, torso, and head in alignment, allowing your body to operate as one unified and balanced system. That way, all of your major muscle groups are engaged in supporting your weight, distributing the load more evenly as you stand and move. Your muscles and joints can work together smoothly and efficiently, as they are designed to do. And when you exert force, whether against your body weight or some source of external resistance, aligning the body parts involved lets you apply the full measure of that force to the task at hand. It's basic physics!

How you carry yourself can also have a profound effect on how you look and feel. Nothing telegraphs "old" more quickly than the stooped posture and rounded spine so common among the elderly. In contrast, people who stand up straight come across as younger and more vigorous than others of the same age. They look taller and slimmer; improving your posture can have the same effect on your silhouette as losing five or ten pounds.

Those who practice good posture also tend to be stronger because they are actively using more of their muscles to support, stabilize, and propel their bodies. Think about it: if you're in the habit of standing straight and tall, you are working your core muscles all the time, not just when you are exercising.

A boatload of studies have demonstrated that strong posture can boost your energy, productivity, and confidence at any age. Those feelings of enhanced power and confidence are not illusory. An upright stance connects your movements to your core muscles, your body's power center. It lets your rib cage open up so your lungs can inflate more fully, sending more oxygen flowing through your system. It can even change your body chemistry, elevating levels of testosterone, the dominance hormone that tells your brain, "I'm in charge, and I can handle this!"

Research has found that when people spend a couple of minutes in an erect, expansive body position before going into a high-stakes interview or presentation, they not only perform better but also are rated as more effective by objective onlookers. Google the phrase "power pose" and you might be surprised at just how impactful good posture can be.

AN EPIDEMIC OF SLOUCHING

Don't you find that people with a straight, erect stance tend to stand out? It's unfortunate that good posture is something we tend to notice as the exception rather than the rule, especially among the older crowd. As the years go by, gravity, excess weight, and thinning bones can seem to weigh us down. Weak core muscles are often part of the problem, and that's a vicious cycle; the less those muscles are called upon to hold us upright, the weaker they get.

Tight, shortened muscles, too much sitting, and poorly designed chairs certainly don't help. Neither do high heels, which can cause serious foot and lower-body pain and even permanently impair women who wear them frequently. High heels tilt the body forward, redistributing body weight and forcing women to compensate by leaning backward, exaggerating the natural lumbar curve and straining their knees, hips, and lower back.

Some people have structural problems that cause postural issues, as discussed on page 112. But for many, the biggest factor in poor posture is chronic slouching and other habitual ways of standing, sitting, and moving. It's all too easy to let those core abdominal and back muscles go slack, leaving your body without a solid, balanced base of support. If you feel tired, beaten down, or depressed, that's often reflected in your posture, too.

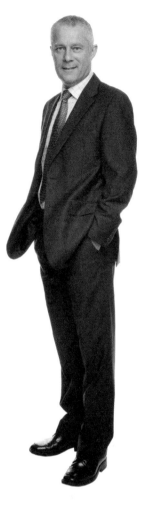

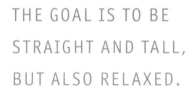
THE GOAL IS TO BE STRAIGHT AND TALL, BUT ALSO RELAXED.

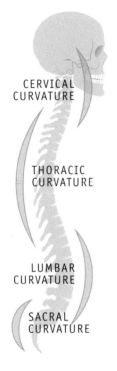

CERVICAL CURVATURE

THORACIC CURVATURE

LUMBAR CURVATURE

SACRAL CURVATURE

NEUTRAL SPINE

A healthy, normal spine has an S-shape with four natural curves, which help cushion and protect the spine.

The good news? With some awareness and persistence, we can change those habits. If you read the previous chapter and know how to make the mind/body connection, that will hold you in good stead now.

WHAT'S THE IDEAL?

The first step is knowing what good posture feels like. The ideal stance is one that lets you maintain a neutral spine position, meaning your backbone's natural curves are present but not exaggerated. Realize that the goal is not to stand at rigid, military-style attention. You want to be straight and tall with your major muscle groups engaged, but your body should be relaxed, loose, and ready to move in any direction. Try this and see how it feels:

- Stand with your heels, buttocks, shoulders, and head against a wall. Lift your chest up high and pull your shoulder blades together in back, letting your arms hang loosely from your shoulders. Note the natural S-curve of your spine; the upper curve of your neck and the lumbar curve of your lower spine won't be touching the wall. Be sure you also keep your chin up.

- Now hold this position as you step away from the wall, keeping your feet parallel and pointed straight ahead. Notice that all of your big muscles are engaged and your knees and hips are slightly rotated outward from their relaxed position. While this position may feel strange and exaggerated, take that as a sign that you aren't accustomed to standing up straight!

DIAGNOSING THE ISSUES

If you think your posture is less than exemplary, it is worth doing some self-diagnosis. Have someone take full-figure photos of you from the side and front as you stand normally, with your feet parallel at hip width and pointed straight ahead. Be sure to wear clothing that doesn't obscure your body too much—shorts and a tank top, some other kind of athletic wear, a bathing suit, or even underwear if the situation permits.

- In the side view: Can you draw a straight line through your ear, your shoulder, hip, and knee joints, the front of your ankle, and the arch of your foot?

- In the frontal view: If you were to draw straight lines across your eyes, your shoulders, the widest part of your pelvic bones, and your knees, would those lines be perfectly horizontal? Or is one side higher than the other?

Are your knees vertically aligned with your hips and your ankles? Are your kneecaps pointing straight ahead? Is one arm or leg more rotated forward or backward than another?

While you're at it, check for issues of rotation and weight distribution. When you stand with your back against a wall, as described above, does it feel like more of one buttock or shoulder is pressing against the wall than the other? Now take a few marching steps in place. Does it feel like you are carrying more of your weight on one side of your body? When you stand, does it feel like your weight is evenly balanced front to back, or do you carry more toward your toes or your heels? What about your feet? Do you tend to carry more weight on the inner or outer edges of your soles?

The beauty of focusing on posture is that it helps you get to potential causes of pain, tightness, and weakness rather than addressing those symptoms in isolation. I'd advise making a written list of what you observe about your posture in the photographs and in the mirror. At the very least, it will help you think about what you've learned about your body and how that might connect with any movement problems you may be experiencing.

This kind of inventory is also a great starting point for working with a skilled trainer or physical therapist, which I strongly recommend if you are serious about improving your posture and fitness. Connecting the dots between postural

USING YOUR CORE
MUSCLES TO STAND
AND SIT GIVES YOUR
BODY A SOLID BASE
OF SUPPORT.

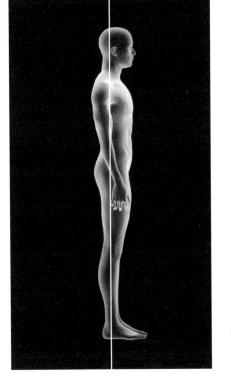
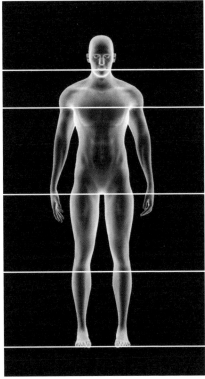

FOCUSING ON POSTURE GETS TO THE *CAUSES* OF PAIN, TIGHTNESS, AND WEAKNESS—NOT JUST THE SYMPTOMS.

issues and problems of muscular weakness, tightness, and limited range of motion isn't always easy. A professional can help you sort out causes from effects and suggest remedial exercises to address your specific areas of pain or dysfunction. He or she may also see structural problems that have escaped your notice. Some skeletal issues are glaringly obvious, such as scoliosis, a sideways curvature of the spine that can develop during the growth spurt before puberty, or having one leg significantly shorter than the other. Other skeletal or foot problems are more subtle and easily overlooked, yet can still have a cascade of effects. Very few of us have bodies that are perfectly symmetrical!

BE AWARE

So how can you retool and improve your posture? Barring structural issues, which may require expert help from an orthopedist, chiropractor, physical therapist, or podiatrist, it's all about awareness. Whenever you stand up, sit down, or make any other deliberate move, take a few seconds to observe how close your posture is to the ideal. Then follow through by making adjustments as needed. The walking program outlined later in this chapter is a perfect opportunity to practice and reinforce your new habits. You can use your walking sessions as regular reminders to focus on your posture and how it connects with your breathing.

Pay special attention to how you sit, particularly when you're deeply engaged in a mental task or conversation. That's when we tend to go on autopilot and revert to slouching. Rather than relying on a chair to hold you up, try sitting

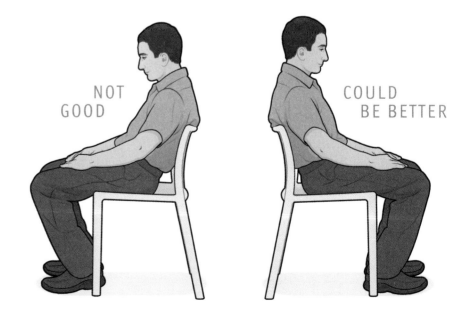

NOT GOOD

COULD BE BETTER

toward the edge of the seat so your core muscles are doing the job instead. If you need some back support, a small lumbar pillow can help you stay in position. Avoid chairs and sofas that are too deep or hard to sit in without rounding your back.

If you spend time at a desk, you could try sitting on a stool or Swiss ball instead of a chair. The way you arrange your work area matters, too. So does the kind of technology you use. Laptops, which long ago eclipsed desktops in popularity, are being blamed for a big spike in neck and back problems because they encourage a hunched-over posture.

Whatever your computer gear, be sure your screen is at eye level and 18 to 24 inches away. The keyboard should be at a comfortable height for typing and allow for a 90-degree bend at the elbow. A little research on workstation ergonomics will turn up a variety of ways to improve your setup. For example, augmenting a laptop with an auxiliary monitor and keyboard can be a big help. You might also want to consider one of the new height-adjustable workstations, which let you switch between sitting and standing.

Remember that it will take some time for good posture to feel natural and become ingrained in who you are. At first you might feel self-conscious or think your erect posture looks exaggerated. But don't worry; in time you will learn how to be relaxed as you stand tall. Don't be surprised, by the way, if you occasionally feel some new aches and pains cropping up. You are asking your body to repattern habits of movement that you've developed over many years. A few reactive twinges are no cause for alarm if the pain is minor and temporary.

PAYING ATTENTION TO HOW YOU SIT AND STAND WILL PAY OFF IN A BIG WAY.

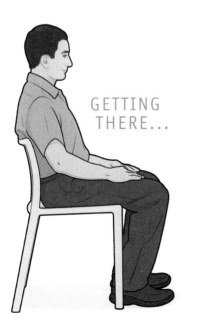
GETTING THERE...

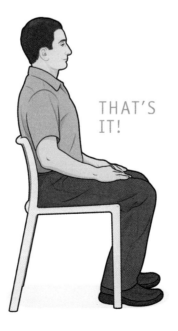
THAT'S IT!

A NEW WAY OF BEING

It may sound tedious to be constantly thinking about how you are holding your body. But once you get into it, I think you will discover that working to improve your posture is uplifting...even transformative. It elevates the ordinary rhythms of your day into a process of actively changing yourself for the better. Beyond enhancing your body mechanics, it will give a noticeable boost to how you look and feel. It also changes your relationship to your body when you are in charge, rather than being in thrall to your old, unconscious patterns of standing, sitting, and moving.

As you advance on your fitness journey, you will find that good posture reinforces all the other elements of your program, and vice versa. Stretching helps open up tight hips and rounded shoulders. Resistance training can make a big difference by strengthening the core muscles that hold you upright. Better posture means better balance, too.

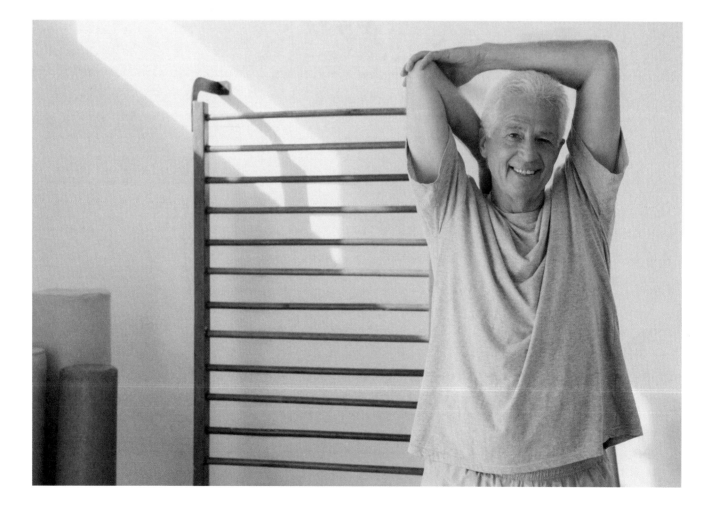

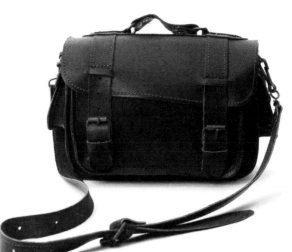

Lighten the loads you carry.
Ditch the overloaded handbags, backpacks, and briefcases, which can cause muscle strain, stiffness, chronic headaches, and even neck or shoulder spasms. Weigh your bag and you might be surprised how heavy it is. The experts recommend that your bag be no heavier than 10 percent of your body weight, and ideally no more than 5 percent. Pick a bag that holds a reasonable amount and has a wide strap to distribute the load. It also makes sense to look for bags that have options in addition to shoulder straps, such as adjustable cross-body or handheld straps.

Switch shoulders frequently when carrying a purse, groceries, or other packages. Whichever hand is dominant is the side on which people typically carry a load. That throws off your gait and can cause signifi-cant asymmetries over time. Remember to mix it up!

Don't lean forward too much
as you ascend a flight of stairs or a hill. While a slight lean will help you maintain your center of gravity, lean-ing at too great an angle decreases muscle activation and can distort your posture. The same goes for using cardio machines at the gym.

Use visualization techniques
to reinforce good posture. Imagine a string at the top of your head that is pulling your body up and into alignment. Picture yourself as a military officer, a Hollywood star, a royal—any figure that you would consider an icon of good posture.

Make use of your drive time.
It's easy to slide down in your seat during long automobile drives. Instead, take that opportunity to practice sitting up straight and keeping your neck back. See if you can keep your chin up and the back of your head in contact with the headrest as you drive.

Explore alternative methods
of improving posture, such as Pilates, the Feldenkrais Method, and the Alexander Technique. Each approach is different, and each has its adherents. Only you can say whether one of them is right for you. Do your homework and ask a trusted trainer or physical therapist for recommendations.

A back brace may be an option
if you find yourself struggling with posture, though they are somewhat controversial. Some say they are a good reminder that can help retrain muscles, while others believe they perpetuate muscular weaknesses, especially if overused. Here again, I'd advise consulting a professional.

THE GOOD,
THE BAD,
AND
THE UGLY

Head
carried forward

Slumping shoulders,
rounded upper spine

Caved-in chest,
protruding abdomen

Pelvis tilted forward
*(increased curve of lower spine,
protruding buttocks)*

OR pelvis tilted backward
(lower back, buttocks flattened)

Body bent forward at the hips

Knees chronically bent
and/or collapsed inward

Feet/ankles collapsed inward;
arches flattened

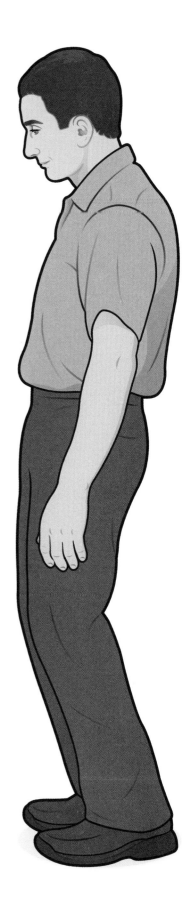

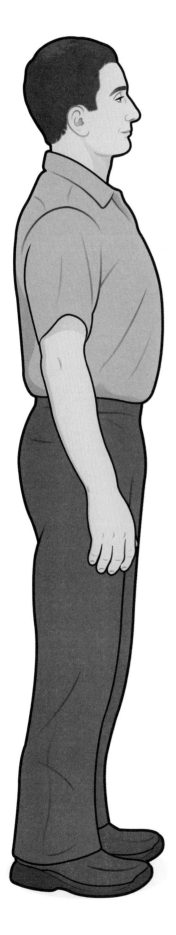

Symmetrical stance; feet parallel, hip-width apart

Chin up, head back, neck long

Chest high, shoulders down and back
(bring shoulder blades together; rotating arms can help)

Pelvis aligned and tucked
(clench buttocks together, pull navel up toward waist)

Knees soft and springy
(not rigidly extended)

Notice how:

- Hips open up
- Abdomen flattens
- Gluteal muscles contract
- Knees rotate slightly outward
- Arches of feet lift

Better Breathing, Big Rewards

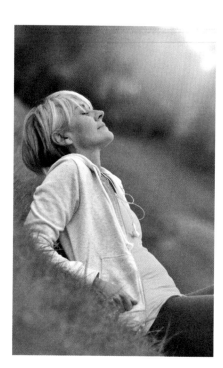

BREATHING
MORE SLOWLY
AND DEEPLY HELPS
RELAX THE BODY
AND CALM THE MIND.

The idea of relearning how to breathe may sound strange or even nonsensical at first blush. Don't we all breathe constantly without ever having to think about it? Even when you're fast asleep or in a coma, the body's autonomic nervous system keeps your breathing going as it continually works to deliver oxygen, fluids, and nutrients to your organs and outgas wastes.

But breathing is also something you can consciously control. If you never think about the way you breathe, you are probably doing it at much less than full efficiency, with surprisingly big ramifications for your physical and mental functioning. Proper breathing also goes hand in hand with good posture; it's hard to have one without the other. Both are fundamental building blocks of fitness.

THE DIAPHRAGM IS KEY

By way of background, it's important to understand that how we breathe is governed by the action of the diaphragm, an elastic, dome-shaped muscle that stretches across the bottom of your rib cage. When you inhale, the diaphragm contracts, reducing the pressure in your thoracic cavity and allowing air to enter your lungs. Exhale, and the process is reversed; the diaphragm relaxes and the air flows out of the lungs. The work of the diaphragm is assisted by the intercostal muscles of the chest wall, 22 pairs of tiny muscles that run between the ribs and help expand and reduce the size of your chest cavity as you breathe.

So far, so good—until we see the effects of our old nemesis, the sedentary way of life. Back when most people's daily lives involved hard, physical work, they were accustomed to breathing deeply and fully. Now that we tend to spend most of the day sitting in one place or another, most of us have let our diaphragms get weak and lazy. Slouching, tight clothes, a lack of exercise, smoking, and air pollution only make things worse, restricting our breathing even more.

Experts say the average person uses only about a third of his or her natural lung capacity. As a result, the process of oxygen and carbon dioxide exchange in the lungs operates sluggishly, so the bloodstream carries less oxygen to the organs and brain. Airways get tighter, so the heart and lungs have to work harder to oxygenate the body. The elimination of waste products also becomes more difficult. Think of all the energy, physical stamina, and brainpower we are forgoing by not knowing how to breathe!

We also tend to rely too much on those tiny intercostals rather than the powerful diaphragm to help us move air in and out. That kind of "chest breathing" is a recipe for chronic tension of the upper body and neck, and can lead to shoulder pain, backaches, and migraines.

MECHANICS OF BREATHING

Because we breathe shallowly, we tend to breathe rapidly. The trouble is, the brain reads that rapid respiration as signaling a fight-or-flight situation, so it floods your body with stress hormones like cortisol and adrenaline. If you breathe that way most of the time, you are putting your entire cardiovascular system under stress.

Inefficient breathing is also the enemy of good posture. A slumping chest constricts the action of the diaphragm and the ability of the rib cage to open up. A weak diaphragm pulls on your lumbar spine, making it harder to move and leaving you more vulnerable to injuries. On the other hand, taking full, complete breaths encourages good posture. A strong diaphragm also works with other abdominal muscles to create a kind of muscular corset that stabilizes your core.

DID YOU KNOW?

ON AVERAGE, we take somewhere between 18,000 and 22,000 breaths a day. Yet most of us rarely, if ever, stop to pay attention to how we are breathing.

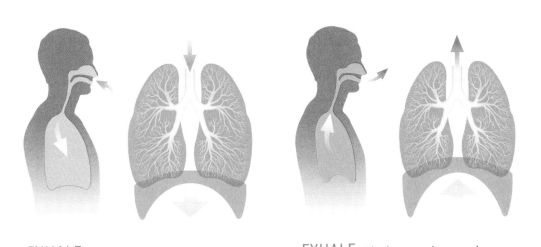

INHALE Diaphragm contracts and flattens as the lungs fill up with air. Muscles between the ribs help open the chest cavity.

EXHALE Diaphragm relaxes and moves upward. Air is released, and the size of the chest cavity is reduced.

WHEN WE USE ONLY A THIRD OF OUR LUNG CAPACITY, WE UNDERCUT OUR NATURAL ENERGY AND BRAINPOWER.

WHAT YOU CAN DO

On the far side of these problems is potential: learn how to breathe better and you will be able to stand, move, and think better. In the last chapter, we talked about conscious breathing as the key to the mind/body connection. But as you can see, there's a lot more to the story. Taking control of your breathing can improve your physical and mental functioning across the board. Conscious breathing benefits everything from your nervous system, heart, and brain to your sleep, mood, and digestion. Here are some steps you can take:

Learn how to activate your diaphragm. Lie with your back flat on the floor, putting one hand on your upper chest and the other just below the rib cage, so you can feel the movement of your diaphragm. Now breathe in so your stomach moves out against your hand; keep your chest still. Now pull your stomach muscles in as much as you can as you exhale. Repeat 10 to 15 times, or until your abs feel tired. As you progress, add resistance by putting a light weight, like a book, on your stomach.

Breathe more slowly and deeply. The average person takes 15 breaths per minute, a pace that keeps your brain and body in an anxious state. Slow it down to ten or fewer breaths a minute, and you will be in the zone where the body relaxes and the mind is calm and clear. Then work on taking fuller, deeper breaths so you can use more of your lung capacity, expel more carbon dioxide (CO_2), and take in more oxygen. Try to empty your lungs completely before filling them again. Ideally, you should spend about twice as long exhaling as inhaling. Exhaling fully is especially important when you are exercising. If you don't get rid of enough CO_2, you will have less energy and tire more quickly.

Work on breathing and posture together. Stand up straight in the neutral spine position discussed earlier in this chapter. As you inhale and your diaphragm contracts, use the back muscles below your shoulders blades to pull your shoulders down and back as you lift your chest. This opens your rib cage and helps you use more lung capacity. Now exhale in a measured, controlled way, keeping your shoulders down as your diaphragm relaxes and your rib cage moves downward and inward. As you do this, you'll see how good posture and good breathing are mutually reinforcing.

Try power-exhaling. Breathe in deeply through your nose, and then strongly exhale through your lips with a "huff," as though you were blowing out a few dozen candles on a birthday cake. This is another way to feel your diaphragm in action. It will also help you learn to exhale more fully.

Keep a good rhythm going. As a general guide, inhale through your nose for four counts, hold the breath for two counts, and exhale for six counts. The speed of your breathing will vary, depending on what you're doing. If you want to calm down and relax, exhale even more slowly. If you want to recharge, do the power-exhale.

Be extra-conscious as you exercise. Take a few deep breaths before you work out, priming yourself to control your breathing during your session. Then gear the rhythm of your breathing to the exercise you're doing. You should inhale as you get ready to exert force, during the easiest point in the exercise. Then exhale as you expend the most effort. One rule is ironclad: never, ever hold your breath, which can lead to a dangerous spike in blood pressure. While there is some debate over nose versus mouth breathing during exercise, I go with the conventional wisdom that holds it's best to breathe in through the nose, which warms and helps filter the air, and out through the mouth.

Can you breathe consciously all the time? Probably not. But do try to practice good breathing whenever you get a chance—for example, when you're walking or sitting in traffic. You can also call on conscious breathing whenever you want to boost your physical performance or unwind after a period of stress.

REMEMBER, IT TAKES TIME TO REPATTERN HABITS DEVELOPED OVER MANY YEARS.

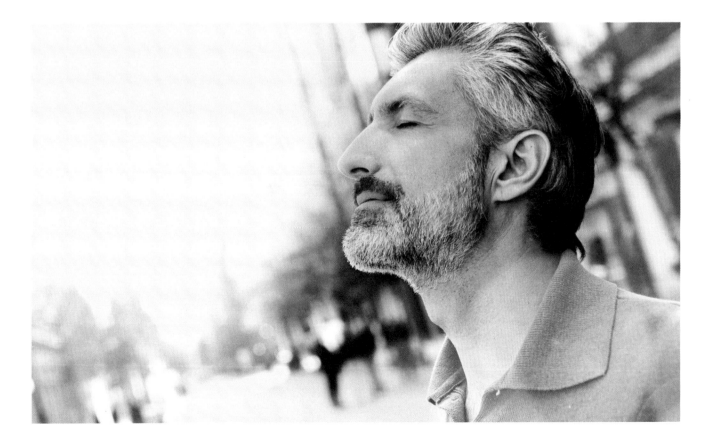

WALKING IS
THE MOST NATURAL
AND UNIVERSAL
EXERCISE THERE IS.

PRACTICE

MAKE WALKING A PRIORITY

My program calls for 30 minutes of walking a minimum of three days a week. I also do my full 30 minutes of stretching on the three days that I walk, rounding out my hour of activity for those days (see page 91).

At first, however, I recommend walking every day you can, for whatever length of time you are comfortable with. The idea is to instill the habit of moving on a daily basis. If you decide to add strength training, the next step in my program, you can drop back to walking three days a week. By the time you start strength training, you should be able to walk a full 30 minutes at a good pace. In my case, it took me three months to work up to that point. It may take you more or less time than that.

You may even decide that walking and stretching is enough exercise for you. If it makes you feel better and more energetic and you don't have the desire to go to the next level of fitness, that's perfectly okay! It's totally up to you. The point is, even if walking is all you do, you'll still be better off than you were before.

Why walking? Because it's the most natural and universal form of exercise there is. It promotes circulation, engages your whole body, and is relaxing in the bargain. It's a weight-bearing activity, so it helps improve bone density and reduce the risk of osteoporosis. You can do it almost anywhere. It only requires a well-fitting pair of shoes. And did I mention it's free?

All this makes a walking regimen the perfect way to start stepping up your activity level. Walking regularly can help you stay mobile and self-sufficient for years to come. Studies by the Centers for Disease Control and Prevention (CDC) have shown that it can also:

- *Lift mood and ease depression*

- *Lower risks of dementia and improve cognition*

- *Reduce risks of coronary heart disease, breast cancer, and colon cancer*

- *Improve blood sugar and lipid levels*

- *Decrease pain and medication use among those with arthritis*

- *Help you maintain a healthy body weight*

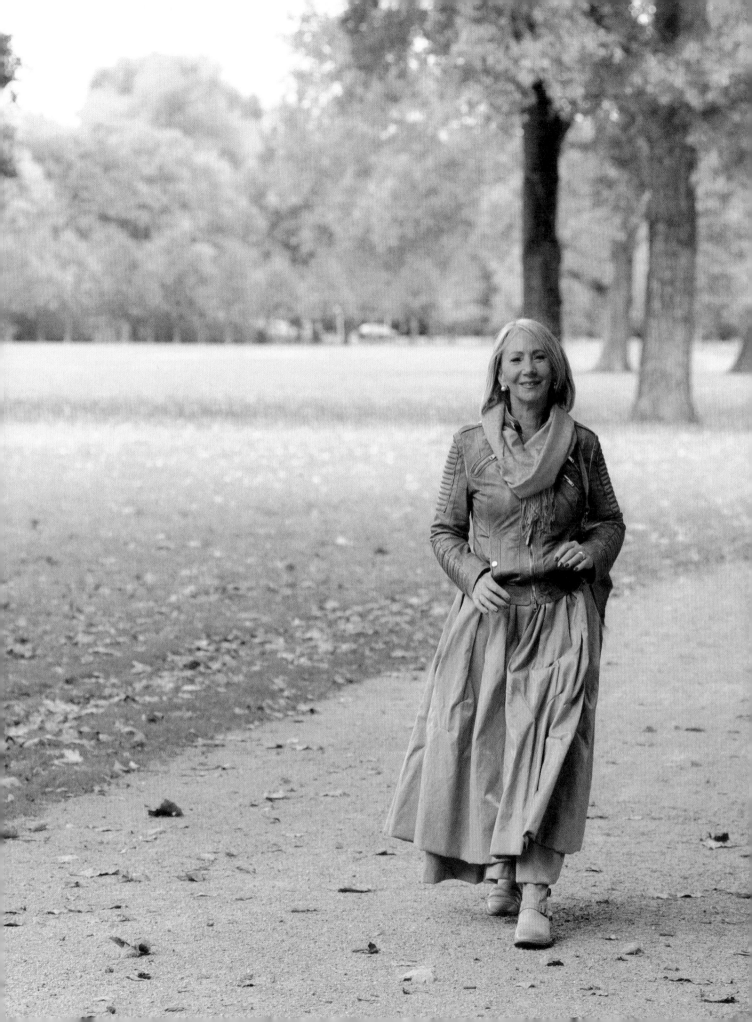

WHAT ABOUT RUNNING

I can't help but feel a twinge of envy when runners dart past me as I'm walking, especially if they're around my age. The cardio benefits of a regular, moderate running program are well known. Running burns more calories per hour than walking because you cover more distance in that time. Studies also suggest that it elevates blood levels of a hormone called peptide YY, which seems to help curb the appetite. Then there's the "runner's high" you feel when the endorphins kick in. What's not to like?

There are plenty of people in their seventies and eighties who've been running for years and swear by it. But running can have some downsides for older beginners, especially for those with joint issues. Running also demands proper form and good core and leg strength if you want to avoid knee, hip, or back problems. So if you're a runner, it makes sense to emphasize strength training on days you don't run.

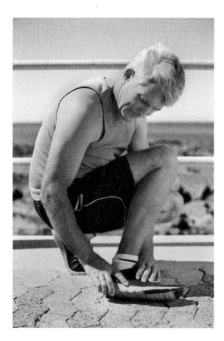

If you've never been a runner or haven't done it in years, don't worry. Walking provides most of the benefits of running with none of the disadvantages. A six-year study covering more than 33,000 runners and 15,000 walkers found that moderate-intensity walking lowered risks of high blood pressure, high cholesterol, and diabetes—three key factors in the development of heart disease—by about the same degree as high-intensity running.

The bottom line is that running or jogging is fine, if you've been doing it for years without aches and pains. But in my view, it's not something to take up when you are older. Not only is walking easier on the body, it's something you can ease into or pursue with gusto, as you prefer.

If you have been unusually inactive, have a chronic illness, or have suffered from a serious health condition, you might want to check with your doctor before embarking on a walking regimen. Otherwise, lace up those shoes and get moving!

PROCEED AT YOUR OWN PACE

It doesn't matter what shape you're in or how many years it's been since you walked more than a couple of blocks. Any length of time you feel comfortable walking—even five minutes—is fine at the outset. Start at a comfortable, moderate pace.

If you want your 30 minutes of walking to count as cardiovascular exercise, you'll need to work up to a pace brisk enough to elevate your heart rate and keep it there. As you gain in strength and endurance, you can gradually increase your speed and distance. You can also choose routes with some hills or steps, which increases the aerobic challenge and brings different muscles into play. To get the most out of your walking regimen:

Walk outdoors if possible. Treadmills and elliptical trainers are decent substitutes in bad weather, but because they involve moving on a consistent surface, they don't challenge your muscles or improve coordination and balance to the same degree as walking on uneven terrain. Being out and about also keeps your routine fresh.

Choose relatively soft surfaces, such as dirt trails or the track at your local school, whenever possible. Asphalt and concrete are harder on joints.

Walking marathons aren't necessary or even that beneficial. A 30-minute walk is plenty, and the benefits don't increase proportionally after that. If you've got more time and energy, use it for stretching or some other kind of activity.

Let your doctor know immediately if you find it hard to catch your breath at any point, or your recovery time after a brisk walk seems protracted. That could be a warning sign of worsening cardiovascular problems.

Find bad-weather alternatives. If rain, snow, or cold throw you off your routine, take it inside to a mall or indoor track.

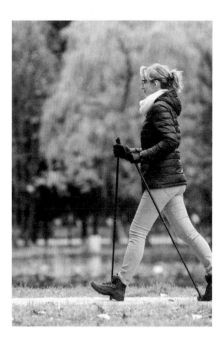

MODERATE-INTENSITY WALKING DOES AS MUCH TO LOWER CARDIOVASCULAR RISK FACTORS AS HIGH-INTENSITY RUNNING.

A COMMITMENT TO YOURSELF

Think of your walks as a standard part of your daily routine—like reading the morning news, only way more enjoyable. Schedule your walks for the same time every day if that helps you stick with the program. Here are some other ways to bolster your resolve and stay motivated:

Use the buddy system. Recruit a friend to join you at a regular time and meeting place. If you're new to the community or don't know a good walking partner, try your local YMCA. Or go online to find local walking groups via sites like meetup.com or nextdoor.com.

Try a change of scenery. Walking the same familiar circuits can get stale. Liven things up by exploring a different neighborhood or a regional park. If you're up for it, take a more challenging up-and-down route once or twice a week.

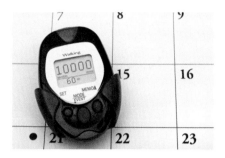

TRACKING YOUR
PROGRESS CAN
BE A POWERFUL
MOTIVATOR.

Track your progress. Seeing how far you've come, both literally and figuratively, can be a powerful motivator. An old-fashioned pedometer will work just fine; use a calendar or notebook to record your sessions. If you're a smartphone user, you can use a walking app or a digital activity tracker like a Fitbit to record your number of steps, distance, and calories burned. Some devices monitor your heart rate, too. Note, however, that fitness guidelines for older adults recommend using perceived exertion rather than heart rate as a gauge and guide for exercise intensity (see page 81).

Enlist a canine companion. If you have a dog, consider yourself lucky You have an in-house walking coach who will make sure you're up and moving a couple of times a day. If you don't have a dog, why not volunteer to walk a friend's or neighbor's pooch? Or call your local humane society, which may welcome a dog-walking volunteer.

Remember, it doesn't have to be all or nothing. Fatigue or overscheduling can throw a wrench in your walking routine. If that happens, try doing half your workout. You may find that once you get moving, you'll feel more energized. Check in with yourself—if you can keep going and do the whole scheduled walk, do it. If not, any walking you do is better than none.

Don't get discouraged if an illness or competing obligations keep you from your regimen. And don't feel like you have to make up for any walks you missed. Mentally hit the "resume" button and either pick up where you left off, or back up to the point where you're comfortable. Any lost progress can quickly be regained.

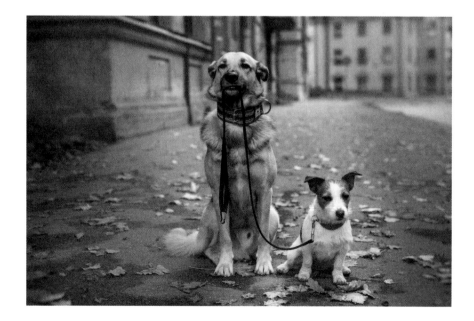

CHOOSING FOOTWEAR

If you want to enjoy your walks and stay with the program, making sure your feet are well supported and comfortable is essential. Wearing the wrong shoes may leave you with sore hips and knees, blisters, or, worse still, painful bunions.

Good walking shoes don't have to be expensive, but they do have to fit. That's why I would strongly discourage you from buying shoes online unless they're the exact model and size you've already tried out. Styles and production runs vary so much that the brand name alone isn't a reliable guide.

Stores that specialize in athletic footwear may not have the best prices, but it's worth paying a little more if you're being helped by salespeople who know how to fit shoes. Here's what to look for:

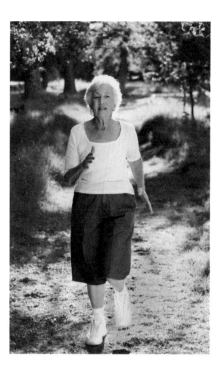

A SMOOTH, EFFICIENT MOTION WILL MAKE WALKING EASIER AND PROVIDE MORE EXERCISE BENEFIT.

- Make sure the shoes have a toe box roomy enough to compensate for any joint issues, such as bunions or hammertoes.

- Pick styles with a deep enough tread to give you traction on loose dirt or gravel.

- Shop for shoes at the end of the day when your feet are more swollen.

- Go for a snug, supportive fit so that your foot is cushioned and comfortable. Don't be afraid to try on different styles and brands, or even different sizes, until you find the shoe that feels right.

- As you try on each shoe, move your foot to the front of the shoe and slip your index finger in the shoe behind your heel. If your index finger fits, the shoe is probably the right size.

- Give each serious candidate a test stroll around the store, noting whether your stride is comfortable and relaxed. Try two or three brands or styles and compare.

- When you find a shoe that works, buy two pairs, and alternate between them daily.

- Don't forget about socks! Athletic socks can add an extra bit of cushioning and wick away moisture, keeping your feet dry and comfortable as you walk.

Remember that athletic shoes change with fads, fashions, and the introduction of new materials, too. As running became more popular, companies built up soles and added thick cushioning. In recent years, the pendulum has swung

SHOES FOR SPECIAL NEEDS

Trouble keeping your balance?
Try shoes without thick treads, which can stick and cause falls.

Bunions?
Look for roomy shoes without seams that cut across bunions. Women who have trouble finding wide enough shoes may want to try men's athletic shoes.

Weak ankles?
Try high-top athletic shoes.

Ankle arthritis or fusion?
Look for shoes with rocker bottoms and a little heel lift to take up loss of motion in the ankle.

Trouble finding the right shoe?
You might want to consult a "pedorthist," a specialist in selecting and modifying shoes to ease foot, knee, and hip problems.

Knee osteoarthritis (OA)?
A new study suggests that shoes allowing more natural foot motion and flexibility may help reduce the load or stress placed on the knees when walking—an important factor in slowing the progression of knee OA. The study found that flat, flexible shoes were easiest on the knees.

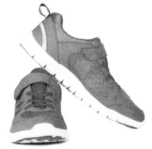

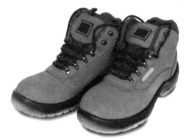

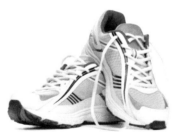

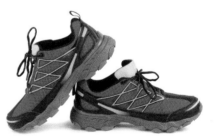

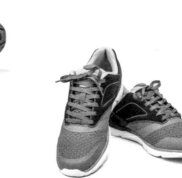

back toward lighter, less constructed, and even "minimalist" footwear. It's best to avoid extremes at either end. You want a shoe with enough padding to cushion impact, but not so much that it distorts your natural gait.

Don't forget to warm up. Doing a few simple stretches to loosen and lengthen the muscles and tendons in your legs will make walking easier and more comfortable, especially as you start covering more ground. These stretches take almost no time at all and are easy to work into your day. You can do them while your coffee is brewing, when you take a break from paperwork, or as you watch TV. I've gotten in the habit of doing toe raises while I wait in line at the store—that way, I don't even mind the wait! Here are three good all-around stretches:

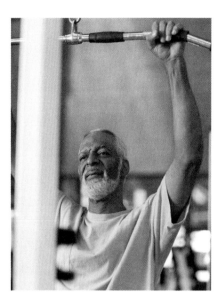

EXCUSES DON'T
BURN CALORIES.

- *Toe raises* Go up and down on your toes, keeping them on the floor as you lift your heels. You can do this barefoot or in your shoes, if they are flexible enough. It's a great stretch and strengthener for your feet and calves.

- *Ankle rotations* Lift one foot off the floor and point your toes toward the ceiling, then point them downward and from side to side. Rotate your ankle, circling first one way and then the other. Repeat with the other foot.

- *Achilles stretch* Your Achilles tendon is the springy band of tissue that connects your calf muscles to your heel bone. Many people have tight Achilles tendons due to sitting and lack of exercise. Women who wear high heels are especially prone to this problem. Tightness of the Achilles increases the chances of tearing or even rupturing the tendon through a sudden movement or abrupt tensing of calf muscles; it's a common injury among athletes and people over 30. Gentle stretching will help ease the tightness.

  - Stand facing a wall with your toes a foot or two away from the baseboard.

  - Put your palms on the wall and move toward it, keeping your heels flat on the floor.

  - Push your body back out and repeat several times.

How far you position yourself from the wall depends on your height and how tight or loose your Achilles may be. This stretch should never be painful. Start with your toes a foot from the wall and gradually move your feet back until you feel a definite but gentle stretch.

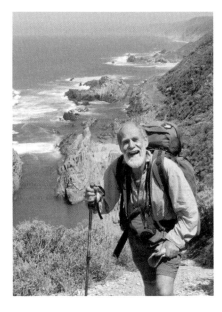

AN EARLY MORNING
WALK IS A BLESSING
FOR THE WHOLE DAY.

HENRY DAVID THOREAU

WALKING MECHANICS

If you sit in a public place and watch people go by, you'll see many different styles of walking. Some walk with their toes pointed in ("pigeon-toed"), while others point them outward ("duck walk"). You'll see some folks who advance in a shuffling motion, and others who take huge strides or swing their hips and shoulders as they move. The variations are endless.

There is a correct way to walk—"correct" meaning the way of moving that is most efficient and easiest on your body. Inefficient ways of walking make your small muscles and joints work too hard, while your big muscles don't work hard enough. They also make each step more of an effort. Using the correct form will make walking easier and provide more exercise benefit.

So when you're about to set out on a walk, take a moment to think about how you move. The ideal is a smooth, easy, almost gliding motion without a lot of unnecessary movements. The tips below may seem like a lot of pointers for something we all do every day. But if you take a few minutes to focus on your walking posture and form, I promise you will feel the difference.

- Before you set out, take a minute to get yourself into a good standing posture, as discussed earlier in this chapter. Now try to maintain that posture as you walk. Think tall!

- Focus your eyes about 20 feet ahead rather than looking down. As you look ahead, scan your route for uneven terrain or obstacles that might trip you up.

- Point your toes straight ahead, in the same direction you're moving.

- For most people, it's a good idea to keep most of your weight on the outer edge of your feet as you're walking. This will help you stand up straighter, reduce the strain on knees, and engage the right muscles as you move. Try it and feel how your thigh and hip muscles respond!

- Don't overstride. Simply push off the toes of your foot in a rolling gait and let the opposite leg swing freely from your hip as you move forward. Do that, and your foot will automatically land in the right place.

- Let your arms swing loosely from your shoulders in a natural rhythm. Your right arm should come forward when you step with your left foot, and vice versa.

- Avoid moving your arms from side to side. That's a needless expenditure of energy and does nothing to help you move forward.

- Breathe and smile. It makes a difference!

Being properly aligned as you walk can help you avoid or reduce pain in your knees and hips. It will also give you a head start on applying good form to other, more complex movements, as discussed in the next chapter.

Meanwhile, think of every walk as an opportunity to practice the correct gait and move ahead on the road to fitness.

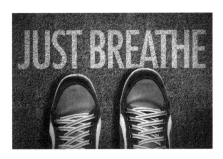

MEDITATION IN MOTION

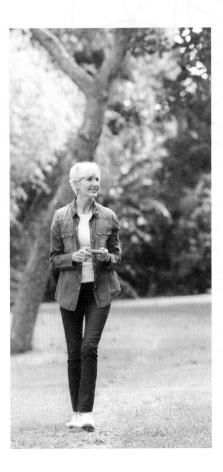

Now I walk every afternoon, and not only because my hips will start to ache if I don't. My walks have become my favorite time of day. They're almost like a meditation practice—a time when I can completely let go of whatever might be concerning or worrying me. There's no phone, no email, no TV.

Sometimes I concentrate on breathing and feeling how I'm walking...how my muscles are moving. Other times I'll let my mind wander, or notice the trees and flowers people have in their gardens, or hear a bird singing.

I meet a lot of nice people, too. I especially like it when they've got a dog, or a baby, or both. Now I realize how little you get to see from a car. After living on this street for years, I feel like I finally know my neighborhood.

ANDREA, 61

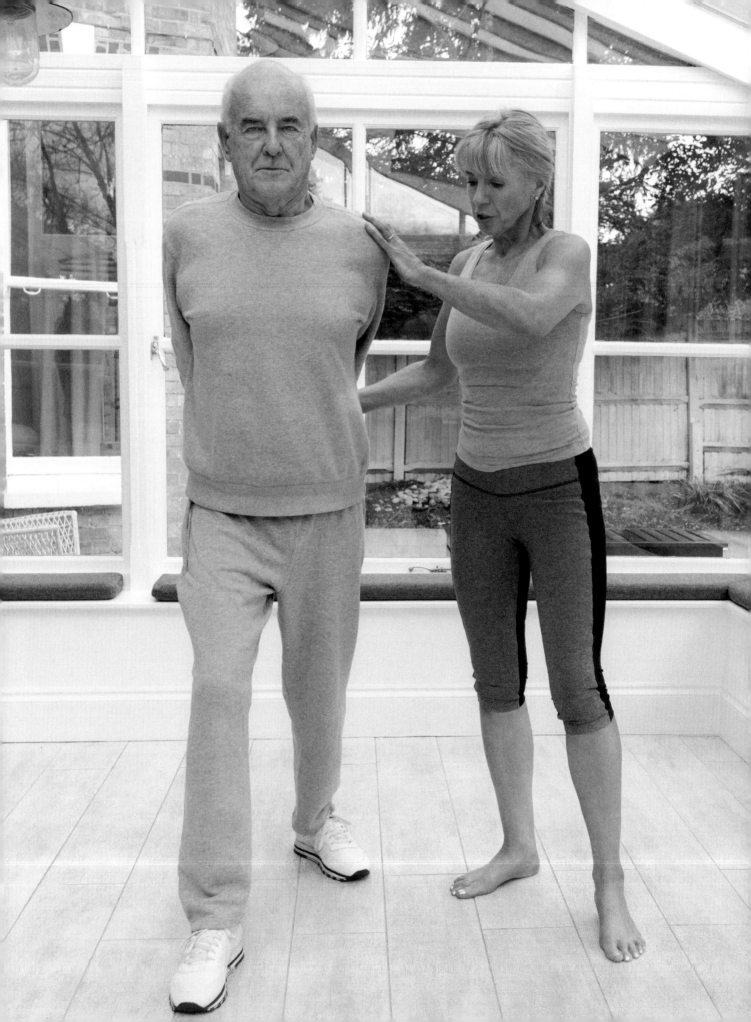

CHAPTER SEVEN

Step 3
Begin Building Strength

THIS STEP in my program takes you into what may be foreign territory: the world of gyms and trainers—but never fear! This chapter will equip you with a firmer grounding than many gym patrons ever have. It will also give you a method of getting started that is easy to grasp and adaptable to your current strength level.

You might wonder why I'm giving so much attention to the matter of workout form before recommending a single exercise. My reasoning is simple. When it comes to strength training, maintaining good exercise form is vital. It is the key to getting results while also avoiding injuries. Having some base of knowledge from the very start will empower you to move forward with confidence, even if you've never set foot in a gym before. It may also help you transform the ways you move in your daily life.

I suggest that you read the opening section of this chapter now, so you can become familiar with basic concepts of form, and then come back to it for reminders and reinforcement as you get into your strength training program. The subject is one you will never exhaust as long as you're still moving. As you'll see, form will keep coming up as you read further in this book and apply what you've learned in your workout sessions. I have also included notes on form in the exercises shown in this chapter.

GOOD EXERCISE FORM IS THE KEY TO GETTING RESULTS WHILE AVOIDING INJURIES.

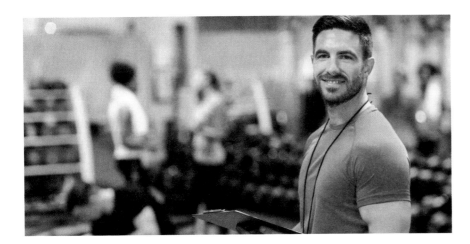

IN THIS CHAPTER

- *Why exercise form is such a big deal*

- *Principles of movement for the gym and beyond*

- *Five basic exercises everyone should do*

- *Sizing up trainers and gyms*

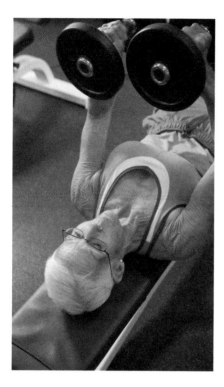

CORRECT EXERCISE
FORM HELPS YOU AVOID
INJURIES OUTSIDE
THE GYM, TOO.

FOCUS ON GOOD FORM ABOVE ALL

Workout books, magazines, and websites typically devote much of their space to recommending what exercises you should do, trumpeting "The 10 Best Exercises for a Flat Belly!" or "5 Moves to a Better Butt."

What they too often give short shrift, however, is the all-important matter of *how* to do those exercises. Exercising with the right form will help you learn better ways of moving, so you can preserve your mobility and reduce aches and pains. It's also the way to get results you can see and feel. Do the same workout without paying attention to form, and you will get much less benefit from your time and effort. Worse still, you could be straining muscles, tendons, and ligaments or even risking serious injury in the process. This is why the "how" of exercise matters just as much or even more than the "what."

A THINKING PERSON'S APPROACH

Let's step back for a minute and think about the fundamental purpose of exercise. It's not just about challenging your cardiovascular system. Remember, that is only one of the five facets of functional fitness (see Chapter 4).

The broader goal of exercise is to **improve your patterns of posture and movement** in everything you do. When you think about it that way, your workout sessions aren't simply about getting through a list of exercises. Their higher purpose is to help you correct dysfunctional old habits of moving and shift toward the ideal form for every movement. When your new and improved ways of moving start taking hold both inside and outside the gym—well, that's when a workout program becomes transformative.

Using the right form makes workouts more effective because it makes them more challenging. Take, for example, a push-up, one of the five basic exercises shown later in this chapter. It's one thing to do a push-up when you let your hips sag and use your upper-body muscles to move your torso two or three inches. It's a very different exercise if you do it through a full range of motion with your spine in a neutral position and all your core muscles engaged. You'll get much more out of doing it that way, even if you can only do one or two repetitions or need to start with a less demanding version (see page 162).

Unless you happen to be a gifted athlete, doing an exercise correctly will always take more effort than simply doing what comes naturally. That's because proper form generally involves more range of motion than we're accustomed to, and engages more muscles—both the small, stabilizing muscles we usually ignore and the larger core muscles that should be driving our movements, but often don't. It also takes more muscular tension to move with the precision and control that good form requires.

The reality is that our bodies will always gravitate to the easy ways of doing a movement if we haven't consciously worked to override that tendency. Avoiding unnecessary expenditures of energy, especially as we get older, is part of our evolutionary biology (see "Are We Just Plain Lazy?" on pages 34–35). It's also human nature to want to use our strongest muscles and keep repeating the exercises we already do best rather than do more difficult ones that reveal our areas of weakness.

In short, maintaining good form *does* make an exercise more difficult than it would be if we weren't thinking about the ideal—and that's really the point. After all, the key tenet of strength training is the principle of **progressive overload.** In simplest terms, that means asking your body to do more over time, leading it to adapt by making small, steady gains in strength and functionality. (We'll talk more about this concept later in this chapter.) When people say, "I stopped working out because it never made much of a difference," it's probably because they didn't understand or apply this basic exercise principle.

YOU'RE IN CHARGE

If all this sounds daunting, let me reassure you. By no means does the idea of challenging your body mean pushing yourself to exhaustion or trying to do something you really can't. On the contrary, you can maintain good form *only* if you recognize and respect your limits. Giving yourself an ambitious but manageable level of challenge is a smarter, more mindful way to exercise because it focuses your effort where it will yield the greatest results. The idea is to push gently, but deliberately, on your comfort zone so it gradually expands over time. Give it an honest effort, and you may be surprised at how quickly you progress.

When you put the accent on good form, working out calls for focus, precision, and control—not mindless exertion. This approach aims to get the best possible results from your time and effort. And as with breathing and

> ### DID YOU KNOW?
>
> *THE PRINCIPLE OF PROGRESSIVE OVERLOAD was developed by U.S. Army physician Dr. Thomas L. DeLorme as he helped soldiers rehabilitate after World War II. His work helped lay the foundation for the science of resistance exercise.*

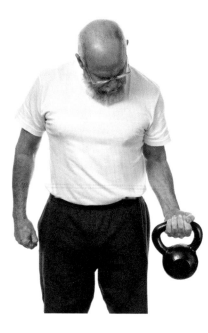

IF IT DOESN'T
CHALLENGE YOU,
IT DOESN'T
CHANGE YOU.

posture, it's as much about your brain as your body. To override old habits, you must put your mind in charge and be equipped with some basic knowledge of body mechanics.

For one thing, you need some understanding of what good form is, both in general terms and for specific exercises. You also need to be able to compare what you're doing with the ideal as you go through your workout. This is one reason why I believe working with a skilled, knowledgeable trainer is essential, especially at the outset. While I'm not saying you must have a trainer on hand for every session, having some expert guidance will help you make the right moves.

It's also true that repatterning your movements takes real concentration. If you are genuinely seeking new and better ways of moving, distraction is the last thing you need. People who take good form seriously don't chat, check their phones, or watch the clock while they're in the middle of an exercise. They are paying attention to what they are doing and striving to do it just a little better.

GOOD FORM, DEMYSTIFIED

So let's think about what the phrase "good form" actually means. The short answer is that it describes the ideal path for any movement or exercise—the one that gives your body power *and* stability because it maintains muscular tension and connection to your core as you move. The ideal path engages all the muscles the motion requires, and none that are extraneous. Think of it as the three-dimensional equivalent of the straight line that connects two points—the purest and most economical motion possible.

Connecting to your core is a key concept here. When you think about it, everything in nature grows and moves from its center, from a tiny bud that uncurls into a leaf to a larva that morphs into a butterfly. It's much the same with the human body, which is structured as extremities radiating from a central core. That's why every multi-joint movement connects to the body's center. Make a fist, and you can feel your shoulder muscles contracting. Flex your toes, and the movement traces all the way to your gluteal muscles.

The idea of maintaining muscular tension as you move is also integral to discussions of exercise form. Our bodies are able to stand only through a combination of *compression* (gravity exerting force on our body parts) and *tension,* the force of the muscles and bones that hold parts together.

The *tension* of opposing muscles—such as abdominals pushing against glutes and back muscles, or muscles at the front of the thigh pushing against those in the back—is what keeps us upright. These principles are fundamental to architecture, and they apply equally to the human body.

Go from standing to moving, and a third physical force—*torque*, or rotational tension—comes into play. Torque is created by the push and pull of skeletal muscles as they extend and contract. Because our muscles attach to bones in a curvilinear fashion—we're not rectilinear, as erector sets or action figures are—you can think of torque as a winding and unwinding of your muscles. That creates tension within your body. Bodyweight exercises work your muscles by using that internal tension rather than any external weight or resistance.

Torque is what gives your movements their power. It is also reflected in the way many movements spiral as you take them through their full range of motion. To see what I mean, pull your hand up close to your chest and then extend it out straight out to the side, reaching as far as you can. If you let the movement take its natural path, your hand will begin spiraling outward as you reach.

When you seek the ideal form for an exercise, you are managing all these physical forces so as to move in the smoothest, most efficient way possible—the way your body is designed to move. What does all this mean to your workout? Bear with me, and we'll break it down into some general principles you can start thinking about and using right away.

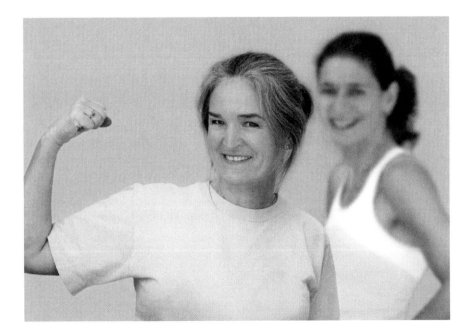

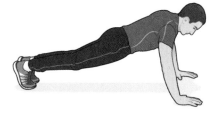

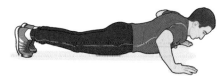

WHEN DONE PROPERLY,
THE CLASSIC PUSH-UP
ENGAGES EVERY MAJOR
MUSCLE IN YOUR BODY.

SIX RULES OF GOOD FORM

I used to think using good form was one of the most important things to do when working out. Now I know better. If you truly want to get fit, form is *the* thing. Yet many workout books and articles have relatively little to say on the topic, generally leaving it to trainers who can work with clients one on one.

While I agree there is no substitute for having a knowledgeable trainer help you fine-tune an exercise as you do it, I believe anyone who works out should know some basics about the correct and incorrect ways to move. After all, you don't stop moving when you leave the gym. Having a grasp of good form will help you apply and reinforce it in everything you do.

I'm no expert in kinesiology, and would never claim that this list of personal rules is complete or definitive. But I do want to share some of the practical guidelines I've gleaned from a number of top trainers across the country. I hope they will give you a helpful overview to start with, and a reference you can keep coming back to.

1 CONNECT TO YOUR CORE

Because our bodies are structured around a central core, there is a natural order and sequence to our movements. For any large-motor movement, the ideal path starts at your core, as close to the center of your body as possible, and stays connected to it through every angle of movement. You want your biggest and most powerful muscles to drive and stabilize your movements—and that holds whether you're talking about a push, a pull, or a squat (see "Core Stability and Strength" on pages 60–63).

For example, you've probably heard the advice to "lift with your glutes." Anyone who handles packages or moves furniture for a living knows those are words to live by. If you try to move any substantial load—even your own body weight—without engaging your core muscles, it's a recipe for straining muscles, damaging ligaments and joints, or even "throwing out" your back. (I should know, because I've been there and done that.)

Another example is the classic push-up. You might think it's an exercise for your arms and shoulders—and it is. But it's also one of the best whole-body exercises you can do because it starts with, and is stabilized by, the entire "corset" of muscles that circles your torso. When properly done, it engages every major muscle in your body.

When you're about to do an exercise, pause to think about its pattern of movement. Which core muscles initiate the movement, and how does it progress? If you're not sure, try using minimal or no weight and observe which core muscles are activating.

Try this: reach out for something on a table in front of you. Now do it again, only focus your attention on the action of the back muscles that move your shoulder blade. Do you feel that your hand is the end point of that chain of movement, and your back muscles are the initiators?

When we do a physical task, our minds typically go to the part of the body that's pushing, pulling, or otherwise changing position. But you can connect with your core if you put your mind where the movement initiates. Then use your mental focus to stay connected, so your core muscles can help support your joints and stabilize your movement from beginning to end.

SOME TIPS TO KEEP IN MIND

- Before you lift or push, make sure the load is right in front in you, close to your core.

- If you're standing, your starting position should be stable, balanced, and symmetrical, with your feet at hip width.

- Move smoothly and at a slow, deliberate pace, so you stay connected. Jerking weights is never a good idea.

DIRECT YOUR MIND TO WHERE THE MOVEMENT INITIATES, NOT THE BODY PARTS THAT ARE PUSHING OR PULLING.

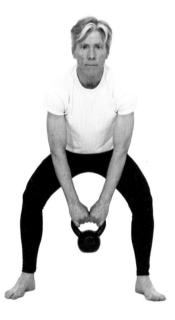

MISTAKES TO AVOID

Bending at the waist to lift something. This puts way too much strain on your lower back. Always bend from the joints at your hip, pushing your glutes back and keeping the natural lumbar curve in your spine (neutral spine). Then your strong glutes and thigh muscles can handle most of the load.

Relying on your extremities to push or pull. You can accomplish the task more effectively and safely if your big core muscles pitch in.

MAKE SURE
YOUR MUSCLES AND
JOINTS ARE IN LINE
WITH THE FORCE
OF THE MOVEMENT.

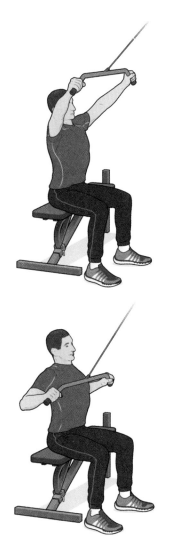

2 STAY ALIGNED

This rule applies in two ways. First, it's important to align your body parts as you exercise. Remember the earlier section on the kinetic chain and the body's interconnectedness (see page 105)?

Lining up all the joints and muscles involved in any given movement enables them to work together. Then it is easier and more natural to engage your core muscles. The joints involved can be stabilized and supported by the muscles around them. And the force of the movement is properly directed and distributed, so you can avoid overstressing joints or ligaments.

Let's say you want to do a seated lat pulldown, one of the five basic exercises shown later in this chapter. You certainly don't want to rely on your hands and forearms to handle most of the load. Aligning the body parts involved—your hands, wrists, elbows, shoulders—lets you harness the strength of your back and shoulder muscles.

This example also speaks to the second aspect of alignment—making sure your body is in line with the direction and force of the movement. If you had to pull a wagon, you wouldn't try to pull it in two directions at once. You would pull on one handle, in the same direction you want to move the load. That lets you use the entire force of your pull, minus friction, to do the job.

The same principle applies when you are moving a load in the gym. You're working against yourself if you jump out of the natural path of the movement or add extraneous movements. (By the way, the same applies to walking, jogging, and cardio machines. Swiveling hips or pumping arms from side to side only gets in the way of forward motion!)

So when you do that lat pulldown, don't start with your elbows flared out to the side. That dissipates your strength and shifts the load from the latissimus dorsi muscles of your back to the smaller muscles alongside. That position also forces you to bend your wrists, making them more prone to injury. Instead, keep your elbows close to your rib cage until the downward movement naturally pushes them out.

TO PRACTICE GOOD ALIGNMENT

- Think of it as good posture put into motion. All the key points discussed in the previous chapter apply: lifting your chest, pulling your shoulders back and down, maintaining neutral spine, and keeping hips, knees, and ankles in line as you move.

- Always start an exercise from a stable, aligned position. Face straight ahead, with your shoulders and hips squared up. Your feet should be at hip width and pointed straight forward. Stand up straight, which will help you engage those all-important core muscles.

- Pause to check for pelvic alignment and neutral spine. Is your pelvis properly "tucked?" (See the "how-to" on page 97.)

- Test your stability by having someone push you with a finger. If you are easily pushed off balance, try contracting your core muscles harder.

- Don't forget about wrists and elbows. Keep your wrists neutral, in line with your hands and forearms. Don't let them bend as you pull or push. Similarly, keep your elbows in line with the path of the motion you're doing; don't let them flare out unnecessarily.

MISTAKES TO AVOID

Letting knees collapse inward when squatting or pushing with your lower body. When doing a lunge, for example, your knee should move forward in line with your ankle and foot. If your knees tend to move inward, consciously push them outward so they stay in line with your hips and feet.

Twisting or moving sideways in what should be a straight up or down move. That's an easy way to tweak your back. When you do a squat, for example, keep your hips and shoulders squared up through the entire move so there's no rotation.

Looking up toward the ceiling in a standing maneuver, like a squat. That can hurt your neck and even obstruct the neural pathways along your cervical spine. Dropping your chin toward the floor should also be avoided. Try to keep your neck in line with your spine.

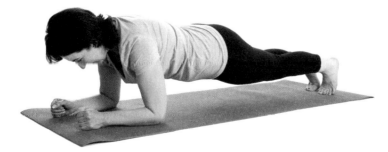

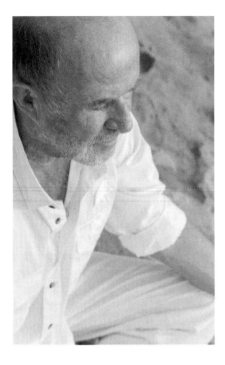

CONSCIOUS BREATHING
INCREASES FOCUS
AND PUTS MORE
POWER BEHIND
YOUR MOVEMENTS.

3 USE YOUR BREATHING

We've already talked about breathing as it relates to good posture and the mind/body connection (see Chapter 6). I'd be remiss not to discuss how your breathing can support good exercise form. Conscious breathing not only helps you maintain good posture and alignment as you move, it also increases your mental focus and puts more power behind your movements.

- Take a few deep breaths as you're about to start your workout session, priming yourself to breathe consciously throughout.

- Take another deep breath before each exercise and repetition. This will help you be fully present and engaged with what you are doing. Inflating your lungs fully will automatically lift your chest and pull your shoulders back. Exhaling fully will help you take in more air with your next breath.

- Sync your breathing to the exercise you're doing. Inhale as you get ready to exert force, during the easiest point in the exercise. Then exhale as you expend the most effort.

- Breathe with a moderate, steady rhythm, and keep controlling your breathing as you recover from a repetition or set of exercises.

- Think of your breath as a power source. As you inhale and get ready to exhale with the most strenuous part of the exercise, picture your breath as a piston that is putting more pressure and force behind your movement.

- If you feel short of breath during a movement, pause to take an extra breath, and try to breathe more deeply. If you feel generally short of breath, consult your doctor for signs of cardiovascular problems.

MISTAKES TO AVOID

Holding your breath at the point of greatest exertion. That can lead to dangerous spikes in blood pressure.

Breathing too shallowly and rapidly, especially after a strenuous movement. Avoid any tendency to hyperventilate, which puts your body into fight-or-flight mode. Instead, take deep, controlled breaths as you recover.

4 WORK TOWARD A FULL RANGE OF MOTION

The idea that you should do exercises through a full range of motion is a "motherhood" principle the experts almost universally agree upon. The phrase "range of motion" is used in reference to specific joints and as a synonym for flexibility; it also applies to exercises. Every exercise has a natural starting point and end point dictated by the anatomy of the joints involved and the path of the exercise itself. Those two points define its range of motion.

Thinking about exercise range is especially important if you're at midlife or beyond. When you work to preserve and extend your range with resistance (weight) added into the equation, you are taking stretching to the next level. It's one of the best ways to counteract all the hours spent in chairs and the creeping stiffness that comes with age.

Yet range of motion doesn't always get its due, even from trainers. Maybe it is taken for granted with some exercises because their range is fairly easy to define. Many movements simply go between full *flexion* (contraction) of the pivotal joint and full *extension* (stretch). With others, the definition is fuzzier.

The "normal" end point for the squat, for example, is the point where your thighs are parallel to the floor, as shown in the illustration. However, some people are strong and flexible enough to squat almost to the floor. But if you're anything like me, how far to extend a squat is unlikely to become an issue. I'm still working hard on getting to the parallel position!

Based on what I've observed, range of motion should *never* be taken for granted, because so many of us fall short in that department. Whether you can do a movement through its full range depends on your flexibility, strength, and physical proportions as they relate to each exercise. It's not at all unusual to have good or full range for some movements and an incomplete range for others, reflecting your particular areas of tightness or weakness.

What many people don't realize is that increasing range of motion isn't just about flexibility; it's also important to building strength. As a movement progresses, different muscles and areas of muscle are activated. If you don't take a movement through its full range, you are only contracting part of the muscle or muscle group. Completing the movement lets you engage muscles along their full length, strengthening areas of weakness over time.

INCREASING RANGE OF MOTION BUILDS STRENGTH AS WELL AS FLEXIBILITY.

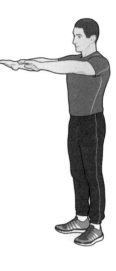

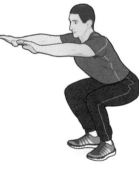

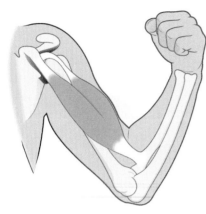

MOVING WITH FULL
RANGE GETS TO THE
WEAKER AREAS OF
TAPERED MUSCLES
SUCH AS THE BICEPS.

Most of us are strongest in the middle range of a movement, in part because of our anatomy. Look at your biceps, for example. It is much bulkier and has more muscle fibers in its middle portion. It tends to be considerably weaker at its tapered ends, where tendons attach it to your shoulder and forearm—especially if your movements don't engage that part of the muscle.

Just as we have areas of weakness in specific muscles or muscle groups, we often have weak links in the kinetic chain of an exercise. These may be smaller muscles that often get skipped as we move, like the rotator cuff muscles of the shoulder, or core muscles that have been underutilized.

Anyone who works out needs to understand the practical implications of all this:

- A movement will always get more difficult once you get past your accustomed range of motion. You get stronger if you push on that range by degrees over time.

- The maximum load you can lift through the easier parts of a movement will exceed what you can handle across the entire range. Thus, there is a built-in trade-off between weight and range.

The first point explains why so many of us habitually shortcut our range of motion. Whatever our comfort zone, that's where we tend to stay. We naturally let the motion tail off as it gets more difficult. And outside the gym, we often "cheat" when we need to complete a movement, like letting gravity take over as we sit down in a chair, or using arms and shoulders to help us get up.

The trouble is, operating with limited range focuses the effort where you're already strongest. It also makes it easier to get injured, especially when you're using your strength for real-world tasks that may require more than your habitual range. You may have no problem lifting that box of books from the counter; it's when you try to set it on the floor that things might get dicey.

Even seasoned gym habitués often fall short of a complete range of motion, especially if they measure strength and progress by how much they lift. But, counterintuitive as it may seem, those who emphasize weight over range may benefit less than they expect. In a 2014 study in the *Journal of Strength and Conditioning Research,* a group that did heavier lifting over a short range gained less muscle size and strength over 12 weeks than those who trained with lighter weights and full range of motion.

Here are some tips for improving your range of motion as you build strength:

- Think or ask about the full range of each exercise before you do it. Start by testing the movement with little or no weight through its full range.

- Add weight in small increments until you arrive at the amount you can manage for at least six or eight repetitions without reducing range. Drop the amount of weight if you have to strain to complete the exercise.

- Consciously extend each repetition through its full range, exhaling as you go. Let your breathing help you carry through the movement.

- Where you find your range is limited, take a diagnostic approach. What's hampering your squat—tight hips, a shortened Achilles tendon, or areas of muscular weakness? If joint pain is the problem, would it be eased by better alignment that gives your joints more muscular support? A good trainer can help pinpoint the causal factors you need to work on.

- It's important to know that a longer range isn't invariably better, especially if you have joint problems or very limited flexibility. Some exercises can be taken too far, putting you into extreme angles that can overstretch muscles or strain joints. For example, if you take that lat pulldown down farther than your chest, so your elbows point behind you, you will be forcing your shoulder forward, which can cause pain. So err on the side of caution and ask a knowledgeable trainer whenever you are uncertain.

- If stiffness or joint problems are seriously limiting your range, passive exercises may help. With that approach, a trainer or physical therapist gently moves your body through a motion without any effort from you; this may also be done with the assistance of an exercise strap.

- Try not to hyperextend or tightly lock your joints in an effort to complete a movement. Keeping extended knees and elbows "soft" and slightly bent will help you avoid stressing joints while still letting you fully engage your muscles.

- While it's normal to feel a stretching sensation or slight discomfort when you take your body to places it doesn't usually go, don't ever push to the point of pain.

NEVER COMPROMISE RANGE OF MOTION FOR THE SAKE OF LIFTING MORE WEIGHT.

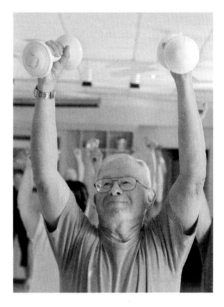

FOCUS ON ONE REPETITION AT A TIME—AND MAKE THE MOST OF IT.

MISTAKES TO AVOID

Not warming up. Muscles, tendons, and ligaments are tighter when they're cold. Taking a few minutes to stretch and get your blood moving before you work out will help you improve your range of motion.

Sacrificing posture and alignment to extend range. A basic squat is a perfect example. Many people allow their chests to drop so they can reach a lower "sitting" position. That wrings much of the benefit out of the exercise. Instead, take your squat only as far as you can go while keeping your sternum lifted. Not only does that create much more muscle tension throughout your core, it also gives you a point of reference you can use to replicate the move and measure your progress in future workouts.

Skipping muscles in the natural path of a movement. This may happen if you use a jerking motion, "let go" of muscles as you move, or rely on extremities without calling on your core. Go at a deliberate pace and try to maintain muscular tension throughout the movement.

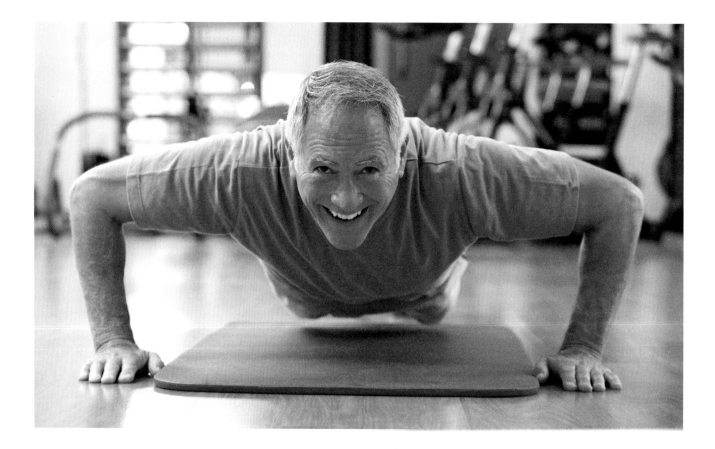

5 CHOOSE QUALITY OVER QUANTITY

Sports and physical training have always lent themselves to quantification. What would the Olympics be without the constant measuring of how far, how fast, and how much? It's in the nature of competition, even if we're competing only with ourselves.

In the gym, too, there's a lot of going by the numbers. We're traditionally advised to do three sets of 10 to 15 repetitions of each exercise, counting as we go. And we typically assess our strength and progress based on how much we lift. But while it's good to have yardsticks, you need ones that fit what you're trying to achieve.

Take the emphasis on weight. Workout aficionados usually like being able to lift an impressive amount. That seems to go double for those with an XY chromosome pair, though women aren't immune to more-is-better thinking, either. It's an ego boost and a validation—a sign that your efforts are paying off. It's also a hangover from the old pumping-iron culture. To bulk up, body-builders typically try to lift as much weight as they possibly can, however they can, even if they can only do it once or twice.

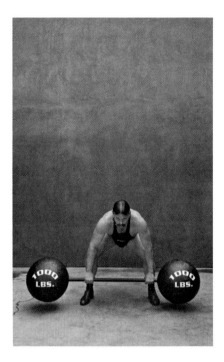

DON'T LET YOUR EGO
PUSH YOU PAST
YOUR LIMITS.

This is not to say that you shouldn't try to gradually increase the amount of resistance you work with as you gain strength. But it's a risky business if you try to lift more than you can really manage. Besides potentially injuring the muscles and ligaments involved, you could put stress on muscles that have no natural role in the movement. If, for example, you notice someone whose neck tendons are popping out while lifting, that's usually a sign of overdoing it in the weight department.

Then there is the matter of repetitions. Doing some number of reps is integral to physical training; it's vital if you want to embed a sound pattern of movement in your muscle memory. But doing a prescribed number of reps shouldn't be an overriding goal. Remember, the whole idea of training is to unlearn dysfunctional ways of moving and replace them with better ones. It doesn't serve that goal if you doggedly keep going past the point where your muscles are tired and your form starts to deteriorate.

Similarly, doing many repetitions of an exercise over a short range of motion can result in strain and overuse because only one part of the muscle or muscle group is doing all the work.

SIX REPETITIONS DONE WELL WILL BENEFIT YOU MORE THAN A DOZEN DONE HALFHEARTEDLY.

There is a mental aspect to this, too. Counting repetitions does help keep you honest. But it also puts you in an anticipatory, "How soon will I be done with this?" mind-set. You will get better results by focusing on the here and now, one repetition at a time. That way, you can be fully engaged in taking each movement as close to the ideal form as you can. You'll find that an hour workout goes by much faster when you are truly immersed in it.

As for counting reps, let your trainer count them, or don't count them at all. You'll know you're done with a set when your form and strength begin to waver. If I had to boil all this down into two words, they would be.

FORM RULES

- Don't increase the amount of weight you are lifting until you get as close to perfect form and a complete range of motion as you possibly can.

- By the same token, don't ever compromise form or range for the sake of lifting more weight.

- Do only as many repetitions as you can do with good form. If it's fewer than five or six, drop the amount of weight you're lifting or try an easier version of the exercise.

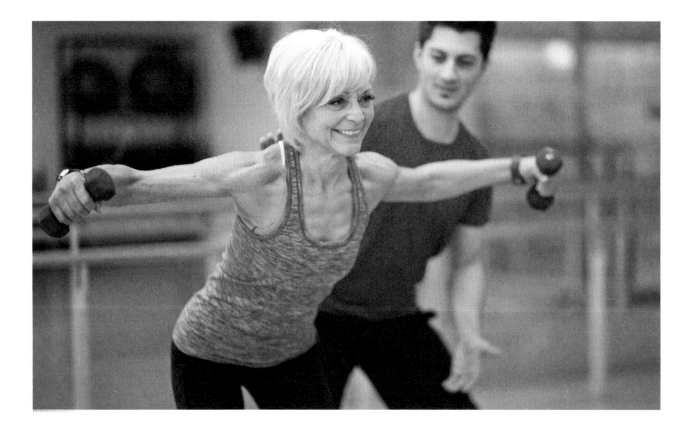

MENTAL FOCUS
WILL HELP YOU
GET CLOSER TO
THE IDEAL FORM.

MISTAKES TO AVOID

Using momentum or "body English" to help you. If you need that boost, chances are you're trying to lift too much weight.

Letting the wrong muscles get into the act. Remember that there is a kinetic chain for each exercise, meaning a natural sequence in which muscles are engaged. If you try to lift more weight than you really can, your body will compensate by calling on muscles that aren't part of that kinetic chain—and that's a recipe for muscle strain and tightness, at best.

Focusing on outcome, rather than input. Let's be clear on the concept: the goal of an exercise isn't to lift a 30-pound weight or squat as low you can—not really. This kind of "end point thinking" leads, even if only unconsciously, to cheats, shortcuts, and compensations that undercut the benefits from your workout. It's better to use form as the controlling factor, and let the right amount of weight and right end point derive from that.

Competing with anyone other than yourself. Don't try to match what someone else is doing, even if you think you should be able to. You'll avoid hurting yourself and make more progress if you concentrate on your own path.

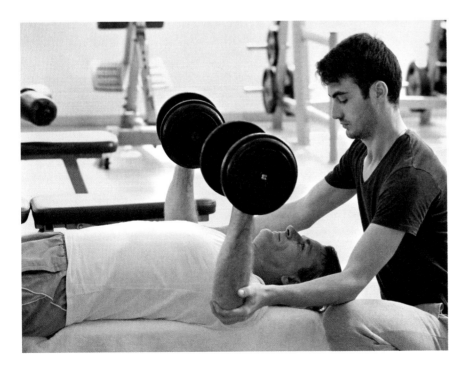

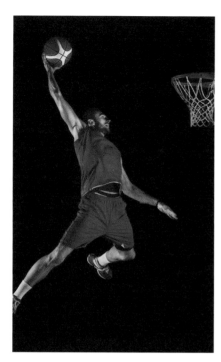

BE INSPIRED BY
ATHLETES WHO GIVE
EACH MOVEMENT
THEIR ALL.

6 BE REALISTIC, BUT ASPIRING

I hope this discussion of form has driven home the point that there is a correct way to move, and an ideal path for every exercise and movement. The trick is to keep that ideal in your sights, and work toward it even if it feels like you may never get there. Maybe you will, and maybe you won't. But either way, you'll be much better off than you would have been without making the effort. That's why one of my favorite workout mantras is "progress, not perfection."

If you can't do even a single push-up with proper form—I certainly couldn't, the first time I worked out—then start with an easier version (which you'll find in the next section of this chapter). If keeping your chest lifted means you can only squat a short distance, so be it. Holding the line on form is what makes the exercise effective, so accepting your short-term limits is what sets you up for long-term progress.

Bear in mind that what is good form for you may not look exactly like someone else's version. Body proportions vary, so angles of movement will differ. Individual strengths, weaknesses, and limitations all come into play.

It may be that this notion of an ideal for each exercise really operates on two levels. First, there is the ultimate, Platonic ideal—the standard of perfection we marvel at when we see star athletes in action. Then there is the personal ideal—the one that reflects your individual goals and potential. While the former gives us inspiration, it's the latter that shapes our intentions and the way forward.

"Be realistic" means you've got to know and respect your limits if you want to grow more fit. Trying to push your body beyond its capabilities could end up doing more harm than good, especially if you're not as young and resilient as you used to be. That's why I'm not an advocate of any exercise approach that asks you to rigidly follow tough training routines without listening to your body.

But as I've discovered, knowing your limits is also essential if you want to progress—and that's where the "aspiring" piece comes in. Remember the principle of progressive overload, one of the cornerstones of modern exercise science? It tells us that in order to grow stronger, we need to keep challenging our bodies, continually raising the bar, so to speak, as we are able to do more.

This means we make the biggest gains when we work right up to—but not beyond—our limits, pushing on the boundaries of our physical performance in small or even tiny increments. I'm talking not only about increasing the weight you lift, but also about intensifying muscular tension, extending range, and generally improving alignment and form.

That last bit of push—the way you give your muscles an extra squeeze at the top of a movement, or pull up a sagging abdomen as you're doing the plank, or put all your focus toward doing one last, complete repetition—makes a tremendous difference. It gives your body a new stimulus and trajectory you can build on.

When it comes to working out, the formula for success is pretty much the same as it is with most endeavors in life. If you make your best effort and give it some time, the rewards will naturally follow.

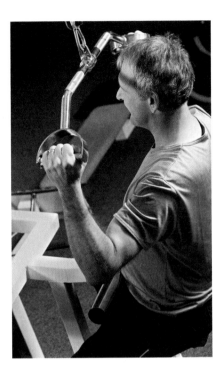

THERE'S A REASON WHY "WORKOUT" HAS THE WORD "WORK" IN IT.

MISTAKES TO AVOID

Being a slave to the checklist. While you generally want your workout to cover the bases (more on that in the next chapter), don't be afraid to shift gears and devote a chunk of time to a single exercise. That extra focus and fine-tuning can lead to big breakthroughs.

Falling into the all-or-nothing trap. Don't give up if perfection seems far from reach. If a movement is especially difficult, it probably reflects the weaknesses or limitations you most need to deal with.

Underestimating your potential. Many people don't even try working out because they don't think they've got the "right stuff" or can't picture themselves as fit and strong. They say "that's just not me," never realizing just how transformative the cumulative effects of a consistent, progressive workout regimen can be. Give yourself a chance and commit to a three-month trial program with a good trainer. You may discover abilities you never knew you had.

Giving up on a workout too quickly. Some of the best sessions I've ever had occurred on days when I was tired or stressed and didn't really feel like being in the gym. On days like that, I start slow and keep my expectations low. I am usually amazed by how quickly my mood turns around once the energy starts flowing.

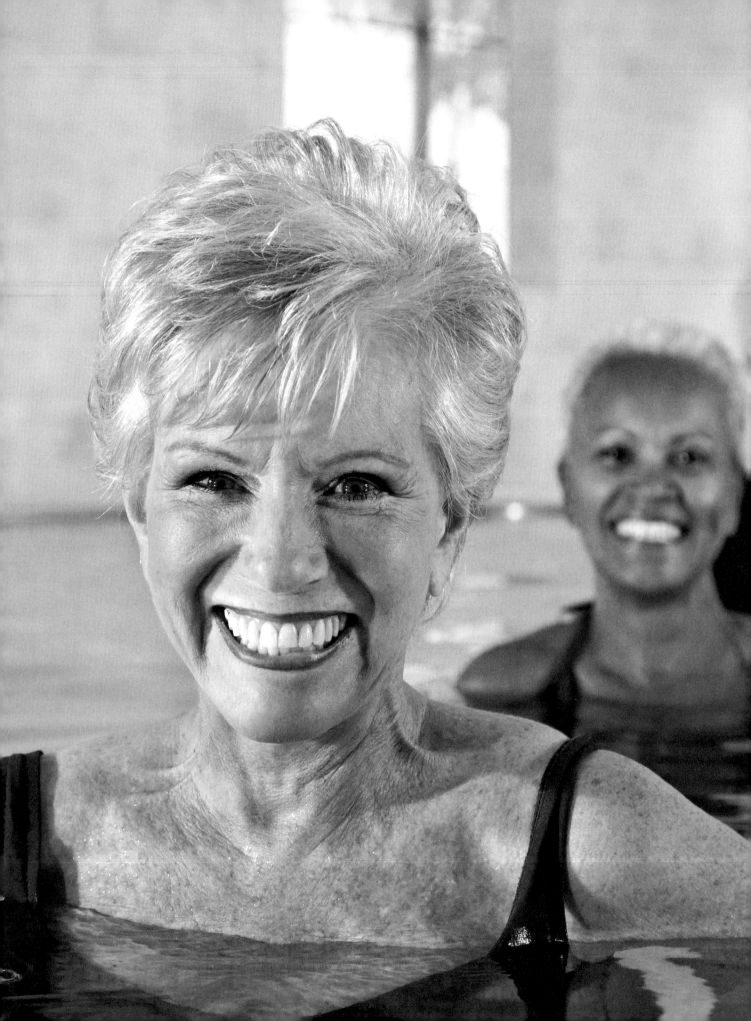

WE DRINK WHEN WE'RE THIRSTY. But do we get enough water? Every system in our bodies depends on it. The human body needs water to enable cell growth, digest food, transport oxygen, manufacture neurotransmitters, regulate body temperature, lubricate joints, and flush body wastes. At the same time, we continually lose fluids through breathing, sweating, and elimination.

By some estimates, up to 75 percent of Americans drink less water than their bodies need. Even mild dehydration can lead to fatigue and headaches. Chronic dehydration can contribute to medical problems ranging from joint pain and weight gain to ulcers, high blood pressure, and kidney disease.

Experts agree that water is by far the most healthful thing you can drink. So how much do we really need each day? Drinking eight 8-ounce glasses daily is traditionally recommended, and many doctors still hold to that. But there is no one right answer, says the Mayo Clinic. How much water you need depends on your health, your activities, and where you live.

According to the Health and Medicine Division of the National Academy of Sciences, Engineering, and Medicine, an adequate intake of fluids is about 3.7 liters daily for men, on average, and 2.7 liters for women. That's even more than eight glasses a day, although it includes all types of fluids. Coffee

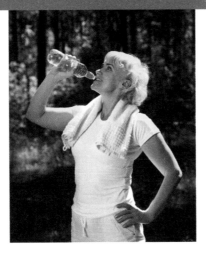

and tea count, too. Contrary to popular belief, research shows that caffeinated beverages are not dehydrating.

Being active certainly increases your needs for hydration. You should drink at least an extra 1.5 to 2.5 cups of water if you do a garden-variety 60-minute workout, the Mayo Clinic's guidelines say. If you work out intensely or tend to perspire copiously, you probably need more.

Look at it this way: drinking extra water can't hurt, and could be good for your health in the long run. Studies show that people who consume plenty of water have a lower risk of developing high blood sugar or long-term kidney problems. (Don't go to extremes, however. Drinking gallons of water in a short period of time can lead to a dangerous condition called hyponatremia.)

TO STAY HYDRATED:

Opt for water over sports drinks. Sports drinks are useful in replenishing fluids and electrolytes (the salts

our bodies need to transmit cellular impulses) after high-intensity or long-duration exertion. They aren't necessary for the typical workout. Skip the sports drinks, and you'll also be skipping unneeded sugar and carbs.

Carry a (refillable) water bottle. It's a good reminder. If you don't find water palatable, add sliced lemons, oranges, cucumbers, or strawberries.

Check your medications. Many prescription meds, such as those for high blood pressure or certain heart conditions, act as diuretics. Take note and increase your fluid intake accordingly.

Alcohol is dehydrating. Alcoholic beverages have a marked diuretic effect over the short term, causing your body to eliminate substantially more fluid than you are taking in. Even if you drink extra water or drink beer (which is about 95 percent water), your body will only retain half to a third of the amount you consume. That's one more reason to limit your alcohol intake.

Don't put off quenching your thirst. While researchers say you don't need to "drink ahead" of your thirst, you shouldn't delay in slaking it, either, especially if you're hot and sweaty.

Watch out for signs of dehydration. Those include dry skin that doesn't bounce back when pinched, dizziness, headache, fatigue, rapid heart rate, and dark urine.

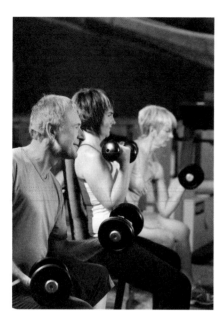

DO YOUR BEST,
FORGET THE REST.

TONY HORTON
Creator of P90X training system

MASTER A FEW CLASSIC MOVES

When you first embark on working out, you enter a realm of unfamiliar buzzwords and almost limitless possibilities. Where to begin? My answer: Start by learning to do just five basic exercises with good form. That way, you can concentrate on learning and applying the principles of form without being overwhelmed. You'll also have the chance to gain strength and stamina while getting comfortable with your gym and trainer.

Becoming proficient in doing these five exercises will give you a solid foundation for ongoing progress. How long that will take depends on you—it could be weeks, or months. There is no time pressure here. The goal is mastery, rather than meeting some arbitrary time line.

THE FOUNDATIONAL FIVE

Narrowing it down to just five exercises was a challenge in itself. My choices center on whole-body exercises that emphasize core muscles and mimic movements we make in real life. Having a stronger core will be a real advantage if you decide to take the next step and move toward a full-body workout. (I left out exercises that may have more risks than benefits, like bench presses, crunches, and dead lifts. Also omitted are those that target smaller muscles, like bicep curls and tricep extensions; there will be time for those later.)

I also made sure to choose exercises that are adaptable to people with varying physical limitations and levels of strength. In this chapter we've already touched on the principle of progressive overload and how different kinds of progressions can make movements more challenging. Even more relevant at this point is the flip side of that coin—the principle of regression.

Regression simply means that the exercise is modified to make it easier than the classic version. Surprisingly, many exercise manuals don't even get into the concept, let alone show how to adapt specific exercises. That's a shame, because it fosters a can't-do mind-set rather than showing people how they can work up to doing a challenging exercise. We all have to start somewhere! In the pages that follow, you will find illustrations of the five basic exercises I recommend, with notes on form and regressions for each one.

MOVING FORWARD

This is the time to start looking for the right gym and trainer. True, four out of five of these exercises require no equipment and can be done at home. Some people have space for a home gym and prefer having a trainer come to them. But although private and convenient, that arrangement has some big disadvantages. It's hard to imagine the home gym that could match the resources you'll find in a well-equipped fitness club, and having varied choices becomes more important as you get more deeply into working out. And don't forget that many insurance plans will cover the cost of memberships to certain gyms.

On the subject of trainers, my feelings are unequivocal. No one who is embarking on strength training, or coming back to it after a hiatus, should go it alone—especially if you're at midlife or beyond, an age by which very few of us are free of physical issues. Body mechanics is a complex subject, and it takes some time and expertise to design a program that is tailored to your needs. Indeed, even the most skilled trainer may need to work with you for some time to get a full picture of your physical capabilities and issues.

As you build a relationship with a trainer who works with you, week after week, that person takes on an important role in your life. After several years of working together, I deeply appreciate my trainer as someone always looking out for me and helping me become my best self. I hope you can find a fitness partner as skilled and dedicated as he is.

This is not to say you must have a trainer every time you work out. Some people want that reinforcement, while others like to work on their own in between "checkups." But until you have a firm grasp of exercise form and are making good progress toward a full-body regimen, I'd suggest working out with an adviser by your side.

You might wonder which comes first—choosing a gym or a trainer? Either way works. You might find a good trainer who recommends a particular gym. Or you might like a particular gym that leads you to a trainer.

As with any fitness endeavor, the challenges of starting a strength-training program are as much mental as physical. It's normal to feel like a fish out of water. Don't worry! With your framework of fitness knowledge, your punch list of five basic exercises, and a trainer to help you navigate the gym, you should soon be making noticeable strides in your physical abilities and your confidence. Take this step into the world of strength training, and you will be embarking on a life-changing adventure!

THE ONLY BAD WORKOUT IS THE ONE YOU DIDN'T DO.

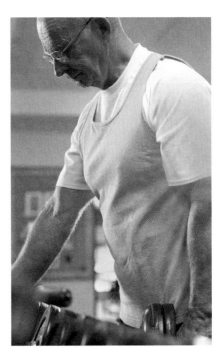

5 BASIC EXERCISES EVERYONE SHOULD DO

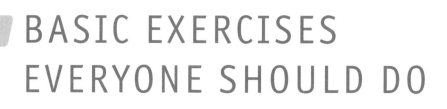

SIMPLE AND FOCUSED—that's the way to start a strength-training program. I recommend that you concentrate at first on learning how to do five basic moves with good form. These five exercises cover all major muscle groups with an emphasis on core stability and strength.

I advise that you choose one of the easier versions (regressions) of all five exercises at the start, especially if you are new to working out or have some physical limitations. You will quickly know whether the regression is too easy for you. If you can do at least ten repetitions of an exercise with good form, comfortable breathing, and no shaky points, or lapses in control, you are probably ready for the next level of challenge. Notes on form are shown with the basic version; all apply to the regressions except as noted.

Don't forget to warm up before every session, so you can get your heart pumping and loosen muscles and joints. I make sure to arrive at least ten minutes before my scheduled appointment so I can warm up on my own; a trainer isn't really needed for that. My warm-up routine begins with five minutes on the treadmill, followed by five minutes of dynamic stretches—ones that keep you constantly moving, such as jumping jacks, seal jacks, and side lunges.

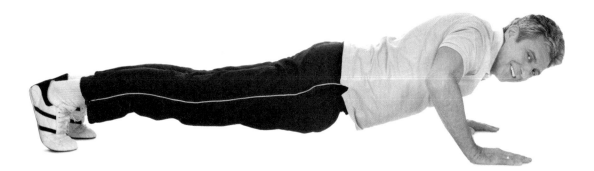

	WHY DO IT	HOW TO MODIFY IT	
PLANK	• Powerful all-around core strengthener	*Easier:*	Do at a 45-degree angle
		Easiest:	Start from a kneeling position
SQUAT	• Whole-body exercise that strengthens for real-life functional moves • Trains all lower-body muscles at once	*Easier:*	Use a Swiss ball against the wall for added stability (this is highly recommended for any back issues or balance problems)
LAT PULL-DOWN	• Works multiple upper-body muscle groups, especially the back	*Easier:*	Use lighter weight
LUNGE	• Builds lower body strength and flexibility • Improves balance and coordination	*Easier:*	Hold on to a support for balance
PUSH-UP	• Increases overall functional strength • Strengthens core, chest, and shoulder muscles	*Easier:*	Push from a railing, bar, or bench (the higher the bar, the easier)
		Easiest:	Start from a kneeling position

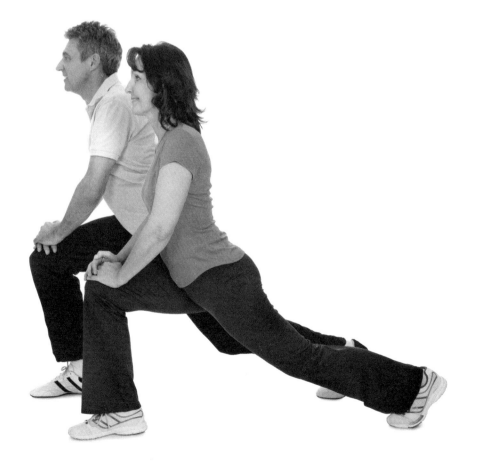

PLANK

CORRECT FORM

- Keep your spine and neck in a straight line to generate muscular tension throughout your core.

- Ground your body with your toes.

- Squeeze your glutes and abs.

- Hold for 20 seconds if you can; work up to 60 seconds or more.

- Breathe normally, taking deep controlled breaths as you hold the position.

- DON'T let your midsection sag.

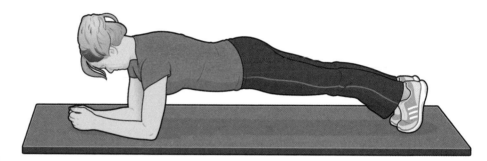

EASIER

45-DEGREE PLANK

Use a bench to hold your position at a less challenging angle.

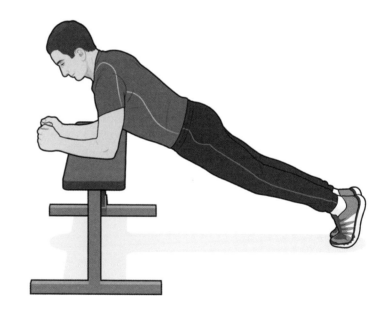

EASIEST

KNEELING PLANK

Be sure your hips come forward far enough to put your spine in a neutral position.

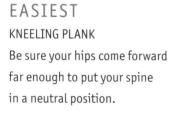
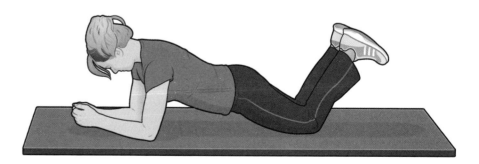

SQUAT

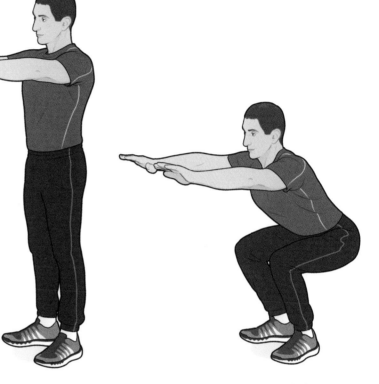

CORRECT FORM

- Keep your sternum lifted as you move (even if it shortens your range).

- Push your gluteal muscles out and maintain the lumbar curve of your lower back as you "sit"—the same motion as sitting in a chair.

- Starting with your feet a bit wider than your hips and pointed slightly outward may help you squat lower.

- Putting a box or bench behind you lets you target a consistent end point.

EASIER

SWISS BALL SQUAT
Use the ball against a wall to give yourself added stability—a good idea if you have back issues or are unsure of your balance or form.

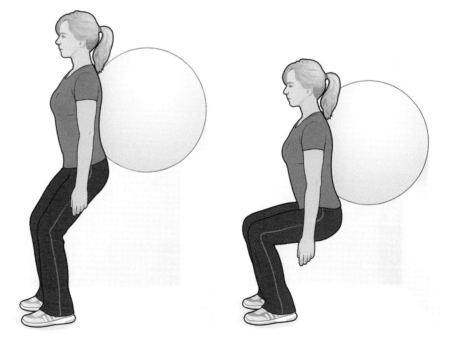

LAT PULLDOWN

CORRECT FORM

- Keep your chest lifted and elbows pointed down.

- Grab the bar with hands a little wider than your shoulders.

- Think about pulling from your "lat" (latissimus dorsi) muscles just below your armpits.

- Never pull the bar behind your neck, even if you see others doing it.

- DON'T pull the bar below your chest.

EASIER

Reduce the weight on the lat machine, which typically can be lowered to as little as ten pounds.

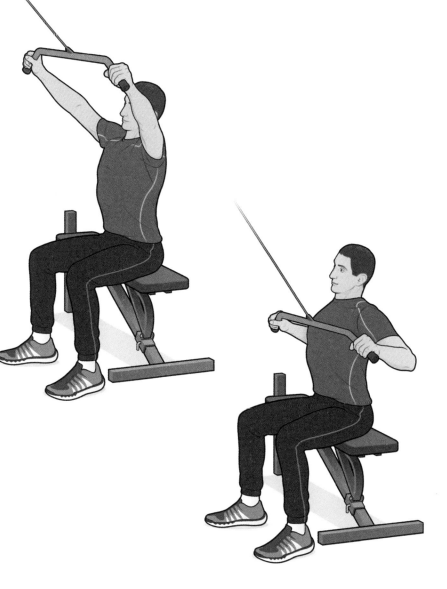

LUNGE

CORRECT FORM

- Make sure your front knee stays in line with your ankle.

- Keep your upper body straight and chin up.

- Lower your back knee as close to the floor as you can without touching it.

- Keep the weight on your heels as you push up to the starting position.

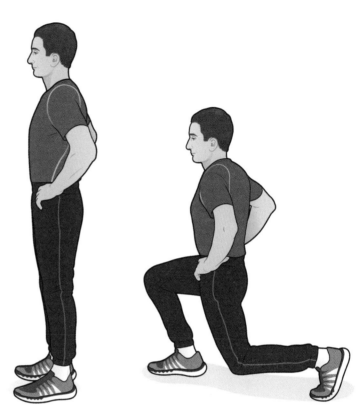

EASIER

ASSISTED STATIONARY LUNGE
Use a chair, bar, or railing to support some of your weight as you lunge.

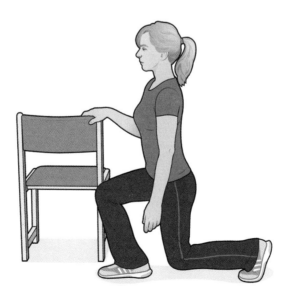

PUSH-UP

CORRECT FORM

- Keep your entire body in a straight line with your glutes and abs engaged, as with the plank.

- Start with your arms straight and your hands a little more than shoulder-width apart.

- Position feet where you feel stable; the wider apart, the more stability.

- Descend to the point where your shoulder blades come together, and then push up.

- Breathe in slowly as you descend, and exhale as you push up.

- DON'T let gravity take over as you descend.

- DON'T let your midsection sag at any point in the movement.

EASIER

Push from a bar, railing, or bench. Gradually increase challenge by moving feet farther from your hands.

EASIEST

Start from a kneeling position, using the same form as for the basic movement.

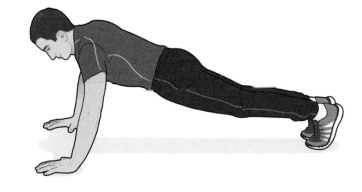

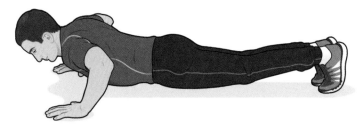

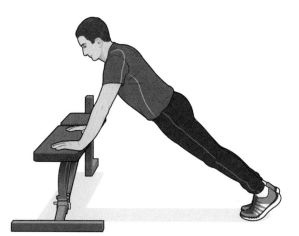

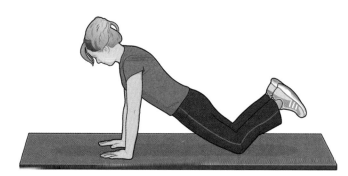

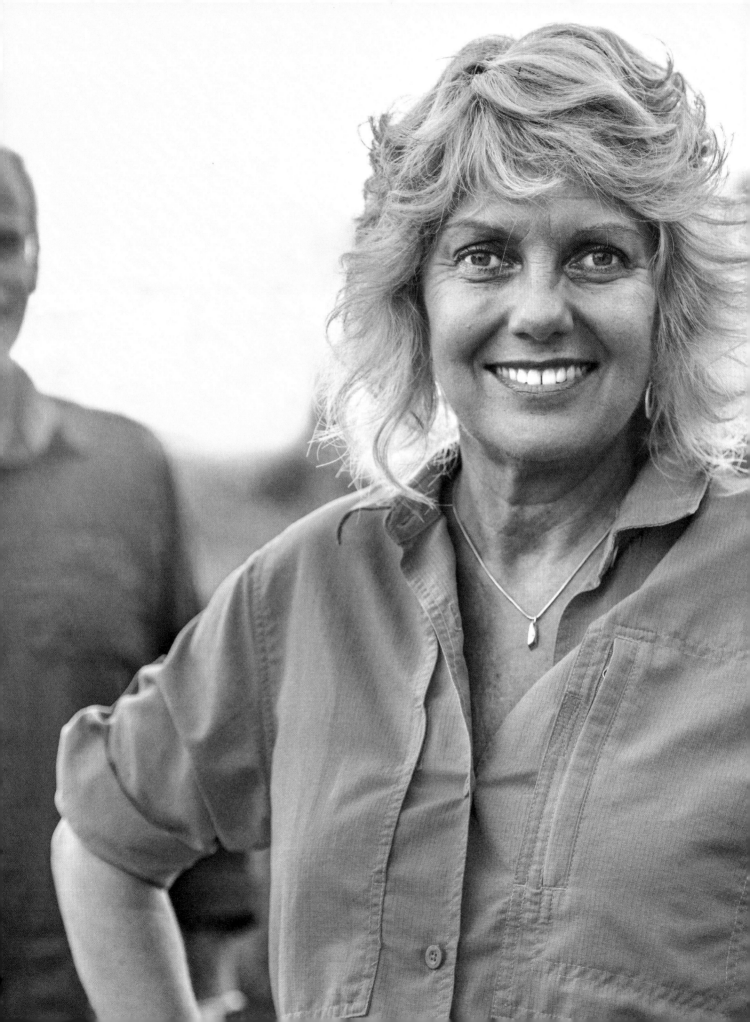

Finding the Best Trainer

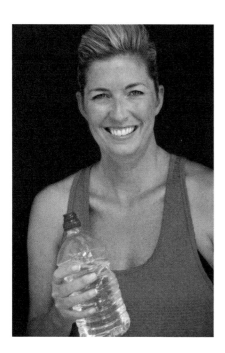

There's no shortage of trainers out there. More than 300,000 are active nationwide, according to the U.S. Bureau of Labor Statistics—and their numbers keep growing, due to both rising demand and the profession's low barriers to entry. While becoming a certified personal trainer may take anywhere from one to three years of study, some prep courses for a certification exam can be completed in a matter of days or weeks. And there's nothing to prevent someone from getting into the business with little more than a business card, a pleasing manner, and a rudimentary grasp of workout principles. All this only adds to the challenge of finding and choosing a trainer.

I believe finding the right person to be your trainer is no less important than finding the right doctor. It takes someone with expertise to assess how you move, understand what you most need to work on, and guide your ongoing progress. That goes double if you're over 50.

Your trainer is also someone you count on for ongoing advice, support, and motivation. Ideally, it's an enduring relationship, as it has been for me. So why would you settle for anything less than the best? The question is, best for whom? How do you find someone who is well qualified as well as a good fit for your particular needs?

Here's what I've learned by seeking out and doing sessions with some of the top trainers around the country:

Look for someone with the mind-set of an expert. The best trainers I've met are not only deeply knowledgeable about their work but also true students of body mechanics, always seeking to learn and discover more. Part scientist, part detective, they are endlessly curious about their clients' physical issues and treat the gym almost as a lab. For them, personal training is less a business than a calling.

Seek referrals from those in the know. Testimonials are great, but make sure they come from people with enough experience to know a skilled trainer from a nice person with mediocre skills. The best source of referrals may be physical therapists, yoga instructors, or massage professionals with solid reputations and thriving practices. In each metro area you'll find a community of bodyworkers, and in my experience the best practitioners tend to know each other. You can also ask other gym patrons who are in your age group and seem to be in great shape. Take your time and shop around.

Screen candidates based on experience and credentials. No doubt there are some terrific young trainers out there. Still, at this stage of life I would look for someone with a minimum of ten years of experience and a track record of helping people with issues similar to yours. Don't be afraid to ask for references from current or former clients. I would not consider anyone who is not certified through a fully accredited training program. Reputable certifying bodies include the American Council on Exercise (ACE), American College of Sports Medicine (ACSM), National Academy of Sports Medicine (NASM), National Strength and Conditioning Association (NSCA), and International Sports Sciences Association (ISSA).

Have a conversation. Ask some open-ended questions, such as:

- What is your training experience and philosophy?
- What kinds of people have you worked with, and what have been the results?
- How would you go about assessing my needs?
- What kind of workouts do you recommend, and how do you adapt your approach to different clients?
- What are reasonable goals for someone like me?

Notice how much time the trainer spends asking about you. You don't want someone who glosses over issues or uses the same cookie-cutter regimen with everyone.

A GOOD TRAINER MAKES ALL THE DIFFERENCE IN THE WORLD.

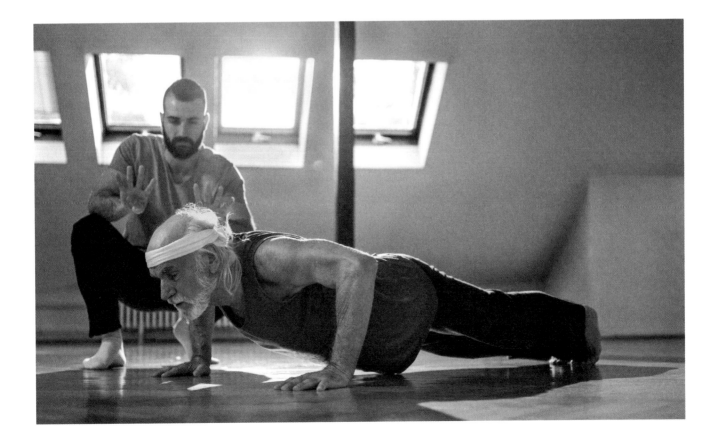

THE BEST TRAINERS ARE TRUE STUDENTS OF BODY MECHANICS.

Style and temperament also come into play. You might be the kind of person who thrives on the drill sergeant approach. Or maybe you'd prefer someone with a light touch and a ready laugh. Beyond having the technical expertise you need, your trainer should also be able to educate, motivate, and inspire you. Personality is no substitute for expertise, but it does set the tone for your relationship.

Spend a few minutes observing. You can learn a lot by quietly standing on the sidelines and watching how a trainer interacts with clients. Is the trainer fully present and focused on what the client is doing? Do you see him or her providing meaningful guidance, such as correcting form or explaining the fine points of a move? Does the trainer keep the workout moving? I'd immediately cross off my list any trainer who seems distracted, spends time on idle chatter, or keeps looking at his or her smartphone.

Where and how does the trainer work? Is the trainer a gym employee or independent? Does he or she work with clients in just one gym or in different places? While some gyms have excellent full-time trainers on their permanent

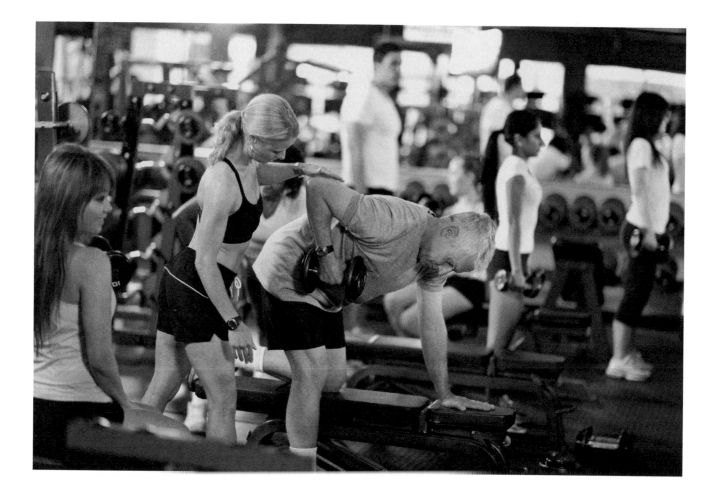

staff, others enlist less experienced staff as the "trainer of the day." Be sure to ask the same questions of a gym-supplied trainer as with any other candidate. Being given a tour of the facilities is fine, but I would never do even a single orientation session with a trainer I hadn't vetted. Trust me, an unqualified trainer can do way more harm than good.

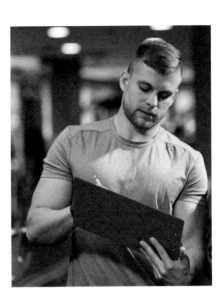

What are the terms of engagement? You may want the kind of relationship where your trainer is with you for most or all of your workout sessions, especially at the beginning when you are trying and absorbing new things. Or you might prefer to work together intensively at first and then drop back to, say, once or twice a week with your trainer and once or twice a week on your own. You may want to consider arranging 10 or 12 sessions at the outset and then evaluating your needs. Be sure to ask about the trainer's scheduling and cancellation policies. Some want clients to stick with a set appointment schedule, while others are more flexible. Recognize, of course, that top trainers tend to be fully booked.

What kind of shape is he or she in? It makes sense to want a trainer who "eats her own cooking." But don't go solely by appearance. A good trainer may not be completely "ripped." Indeed, someone who looks like an action figure may be more geared to the old bodybuilding culture than to functional fitness. Some of the fittest people I've ever met don't stand out from a crowd until you see them in action. In short, good trainers come in different shapes and sizes. It's what they know and how they work with you that counts.

Don't base your decision on cost alone. Prices for personal training vary widely; certified trainers may charge anywhere from $50 an hour in low-cost areas to $100 or $150 an hour in more expensive markets. As with other professional services, cost may not be a reliable indicator of quality. And don't forget that you can pare the costs of training by sharing your sessions with a partner or friend, and maybe have more fun in the process.

Be a good client. Don't treat your trainer like some anonymous service provider; he or she is a skilled professional whose time is valuable and who deserves to be treated with respect. That means showing up on time for appointments, paying on time for each session, and never canceling at the last minute for some trivial reason (e.g., "I don't feel like working out today"). It's also important that you honor your shared commitment by staying focused and making a genuine effort during your workout. If you make an honest effort, and are willing to push on your limits in order to progress, then you, too, will get the best your trainer has to offer.

Which Gym to Choose?

Gyms abound, and they can vary greatly in their offerings and orientation. Personally, I am more impressed by state-of-the-art equipment and knowledgeable training staff than by accoutrements such as plush towels, brass-fitted lockers, and juice bars. But you may find value in amenities such as saunas, swimming pools, on-site massage therapists and nutritionists, and indoor jogging tracks. Many gyms also offer a variety of fitness classes, which may be included in your membership or carry a separate charge. Then there is the feel of the place—the mix of patrons, the layout, and even the volume of the music.

When you're checking out a gym, it makes sense to go at the times you're most likely to use it. Many get crowded in the early morning and at the end of the workday, but are much less busy at other times. Don't stop with the membership department; talk with the training director, if at all possible, about what the gym offers someone with your needs and preferences. Think about what's important to you, check online reviews, and don't be afraid to take your time and shop around before making a decision.

Here's a checklist of things I look for in a gym:

☐ An emphasis on functional fitness and multifaceted strength training and conditioning for adults of all ages. I avoid gyms that are geared mainly to competitive bodybuilders or are tied to a single proprietary training approach.

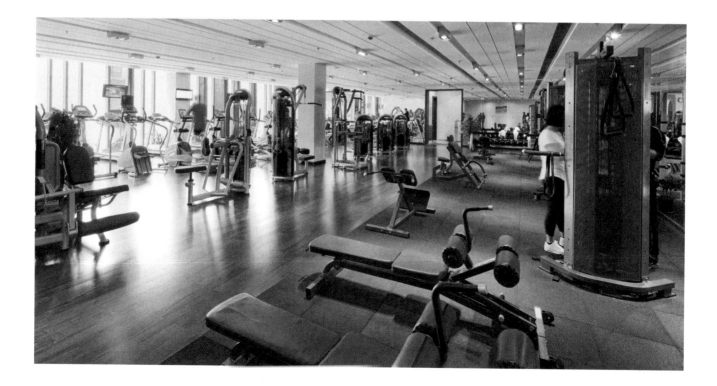

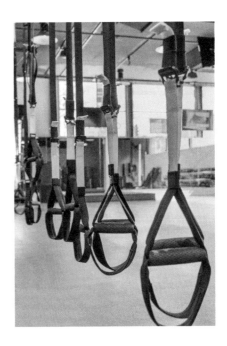

- [ ] A full array of free weights (dumbbells, barbells, and weight plates), weight racks, and benches

- [ ] Several cable machines

- [ ] Ample space for stretching and warm-ups (this is important!)

- [ ] Up-to-date cardio machines—while every piece of equipment may not be brand-new, the gym should have some higher-tech gear such as elliptical trainers, stair-climbers, or ergonomic rowers. It should also have some recumbent stationary bikes, which some people find more comfortable and easier on joints, as well as upright models.

- [ ] A full complement of training aids such as exercise mats, foam rollers, Bosus, Swiss balls, medicine balls, resistance bands, TRX straps, Pilates reformers, battle ropes, ViPRs, and weighted vests

- [ ] Policies that allow clients to work with independent trainers rather than limit you to those employed by the gym

- [ ] Clean, well-maintained gym floor, showers, and locker rooms

- [ ] Staff that is courteous and trained in emergency procedures

- [ ] A location close enough that travel time and traffic won't get in the way of your workouts

IT'S ENERGIZING TO BE AROUND OTHER PEOPLE WHO ARE WORKING HARD TO BECOME FIT.

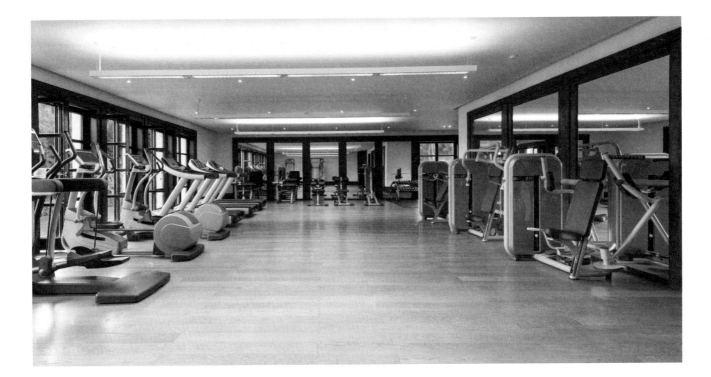

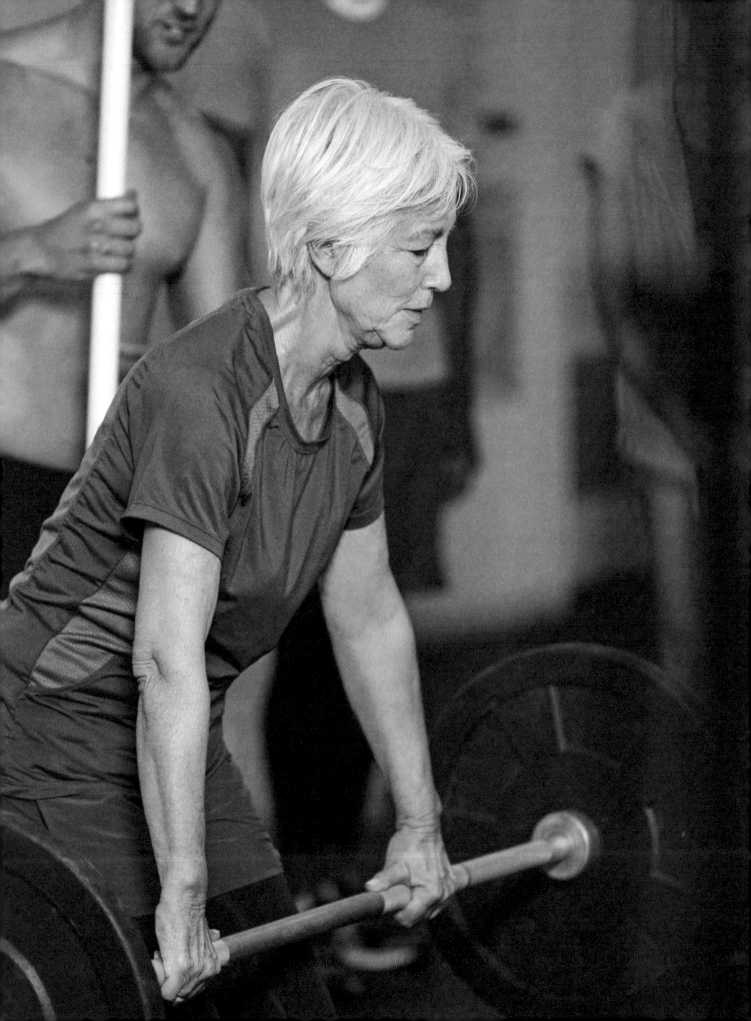

CHAPTER EIGHT

Step 4
Advance to a Full-Body Workout

SURPRISING AS IT MAY SEEM, if you have mastered some version of the five basic exercises in the previous chapter and can do them with reasonably good form, the toughest part is over. Once you have added regular strength training to your stretching and walking disciplines, you are well on the path to lifelong fitness.

This chapter is all about how you can stay active and keep progressing for years to come. Why am I putting so much emphasis on the notion of continuing progress? It's partly a matter of being realistic. Once you hit your sixties or seventies, you realize that your body doesn't stay the same for very long. The process of aging is occurring at the genetic and cellular levels, and what we see in the mirror are only the outward signs. Sooner or later we all feel other subtle and not-so-subtle manifestations of age. Even if you're in pretty good shape, you may notice a few more aches and pains, a little more stiffness when getting up from a chair, and maybe a little less energy than we had when youngsters of 40 or 45. Working at fitness when you're older is like kayaking upstream. You have to paddle just to stay in place, and paddle a little harder if you want to get somewhere.

THERE IS ALWAYS
FEAR IN GOING
SOMEWHERE NEW...
BUT FEAR CAN
TURN TO JOY.

YO-YO MA

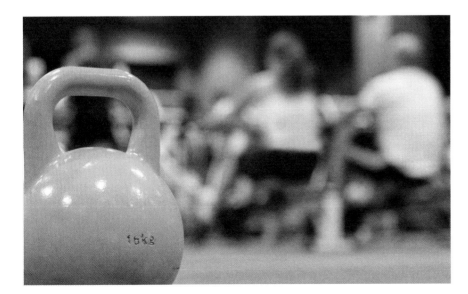

IN THIS CHAPTER

- *How to train smarter, not harder*

- *Keys to making progress without pain*

- *Five basic exercises, taken to the next level*

- *A customizable workout template*

- *Finding the joy*

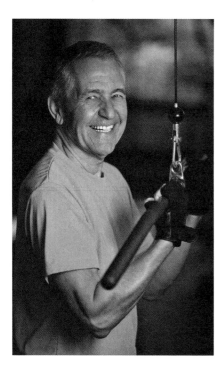

A LITTLE PROGRESS
EACH WEEK ADDS UP
TO BIG RESULTS.

But here's what people don't know when they're just starting to work out: while getting fit can be hard, staying fit is a lot of fun! There is always something else to learn, something new to try. The secret is to add variety and keep giving yourself new challenges that are just beyond your comfort level, but not out of reach. Meeting those challenges is a reward in itself, not unlike the feeling of triumph you get from solving a complicated puzzle or executing a perfect golf shot. Then there's the very real sense of confidence and power you gain by pushing back against the forces of time and gravity. Listen to the inner voice that says, "If I can do that...what else can I do?" It may inspire you to flex other kinds of muscles—the ones that open up new creative pursuits and fresh ways of looking at the world.

This chapter offers principles that I hope will empower you to keep advancing in your fitness journey, and enjoy the ride! One of the gifts of age is a keener appreciation for the simple joys of life lost to those who are no longer able to go for a long walk, pick up a grandchild, or take care of their own daily needs. Once you realize that being physically fit is the Great Enabler—the nonnegotiable prerequisite for your continuing freedom, independence, and quality of life as the years go by—then walking, stretching, and strength training feel less like chores and more like opportunities to enrich your life. Be grateful for your body and what it can do. Whatever the mix of fitness activities you pursue, think of them as your personal recipe for a feel-good potion that no amount of money can buy.

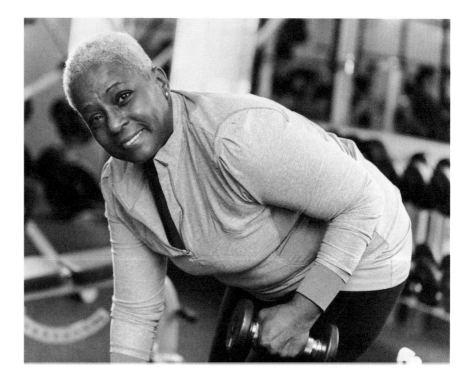

FIND MULTIPLE WAYS TO PROGRESS

One of the most renowned athletes of ancient Greece was Milo of Croton, a real-life wrestler who inspired fantastic tales of superhuman strength and power. As legend has it, his training began in childhood when his father gave him a newborn calf. Every day after doing his chores, Milo would put the calf on his shoulders and walk down to the village square and back. As time went on and the calf grew, Milo kept up his training, until eventually he was able to carry a full-size ox on his back. He went on to become the most revered wrestler in the ancient world, winning the championship at six Olympic Games and seven Pythian Games.

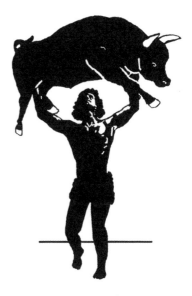

MILO OF CROTON

CONSIDER THE OPTIONS

Many people who want to get stronger assume they should use the same approach Milo did—that is, continually increase the amount of weight they lift when working out. That is certainly one way to progress, but there are many other ways to turn up the dial on an exercise. It makes sense to consider those options before you try lifting more weight, especially if you haven't yet achieved good form or a complete range of motion.

Below are a variety of techniques to add challenge to an exercise. One of them, trying different and more advanced versions, is highlighted in this chapter. But no matter what techniques you use, commonsense cautions apply:

- **Be selective.** You don't have to advance multiple exercises at the same time. It makes more sense to work on one exercise or one part of the body at a time. You'll avoid getting overly fatigued and will be able to see exactly how your body reacts to each change.

- **Add challenge gradually.** Don't take or try to make big leaps too quickly.

- **Don't be in denial about your physical issues and weaknesses.** Adapting for them is a much better approach (read more on that below).

- **Keep ego out of it.** Don't get carried away by a desire to match someone else or some arbitrary benchmark.

Seven Ways to Progress

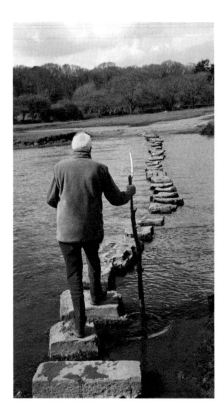

THE ULTIMATE
WORKOUT RULE:
BE PRESENT.

I won't claim that this list is exhaustive, but I hope it will inspire you to be creative and use a variety of approaches as you advance in your training.

1 **Improve exercise form.** As far as I'm concerned, this is always the place to start advancing an exercise. As was discussed in Chapter 7, doing an exercise correctly will always be more difficult than doing it with an indifference to form. When doing a squat, for example, it's surprising how much internal muscular resistance you can create simply by lifting your sternum and holding that line as you move.

Exercise sets traditionally consist of 10 to 15 repetitions. Start with 10 reps and gradually work up to 15. When you can do 15 reps with good form, add some weight and drop back to 10 reps.

2 **Increase range of motion.** I am a big advocate of striving for a full range of motion in whatever exercise you do. Even if you don't achieve it right away, your progress toward it will help you strengthen areas of muscle that might otherwise be overlooked.

3 **Do more advanced versions of an exercise.** You'll see five pages of examples and more discussion of this approach below. Even if an exercise variation isn't inherently more difficult, you may find it more challenging if it engages muscles you don't frequently use.

4 **Make the exercise unilateral.** In other words, do the exercise on one side of the body at a time, as you would with a single-arm dumbbell press or row. Unilateral exercises can build strength rapidly. They are more demanding than bilateral movements because they not only focus effort on one side of the body, but also call upon your core muscles to help stabilize and balance your body as you move. In fact, I'd say that most unilateral exercises also check the box in the core category if you do them properly. Another consideration: unilateral movements will immediately reveal imbalances in strength. They will also help you even out those asymmetries over time. This can be helpful, since most of us tend to rely on one side of the body more than on the other.

5 **Use different equipment.** Any good gym has a variety of workout gear, and there are trade-offs with each choice (see page 175). I tend to be more of a fan of free weights and bodyweight exercises than exercise machines, which I generally find too restrictive. Still, because machines dictate the path of a movement (as with the lat pulldown), they can sometimes make it easier to achieve correct form.

What Kind of Equipment to Choose?

*There is no one "best" answer,
and you may well want to use a mix*

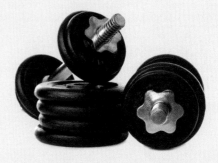

	PROS	CONS
FREE WEIGHTS *Dumbbells, barbells, kettlebells*	• Versatile and flexible • Mimic functional movements • Engage more muscles • Can be used unilaterally for added challenge • Good for extending range	• Higher risk of injury unless proper form is used
CABLES *Weight stacks in many different configurations*	• Highly versatile and flexible • Allow full range of movement • Weight can be added in small increments	• Good form is required to do movements safely and effectively so you need to get the angles right
BODYWEIGHT EXERCISES *Use internal muscular tension to lift some portion of your body's weight*	• Mimic functional movements • Efficient—multiple muscles and joints are engaged • Can be done anywhere	• Don't apply to every kind of exercise • Ability to increase weight (progressive overload) is somewhat limited
EXERCISE MACHINES *Designed around a single muscle or muscle group*	• Exercise path is dictated • Usually target specific muscles • May help you lift more weight • Weight can be added in small increments	• Movement is restricted to one or two planes • Range may not be complete • Isolating muscles is less efficient • Not all are well designed • Some risk of injury due to repetitive movement

IMAGINE YOURSELF
SIX MONTHS FROM NOW.

6 **See how many reps you can do within a given time.** For example, how many push-ups can you do in 60 seconds? If you want to torch some calories as you build strength, this is one way to do it.

7 **Slow things down.** Almost any exercise becomes more challenging if you drop the speed with which you do it. When you advance to the point where you can easily knock out a few push-ups, try doing them at a reduced tempo and you'll see what I mean. You can also do what are called "negatives." Most exercises have two phases—the lowering phase, in which you go from the starting to the lifting position, and the lifting phase, in which you exert the most effort. When you do negatives, you substantially slow down the lowering phase, so you are actively fighting gravity and resisting the pull of the weight. Similarly, you can get an assist in the lifting phase— for example, enlist your trainer or use a resistance band to give you some help at the point where you can't entirely lift the weight yourself—and then forgo the assist in the lowering phase, where gravity is on your side. When used sensibly, negatives can give your training a real boost.

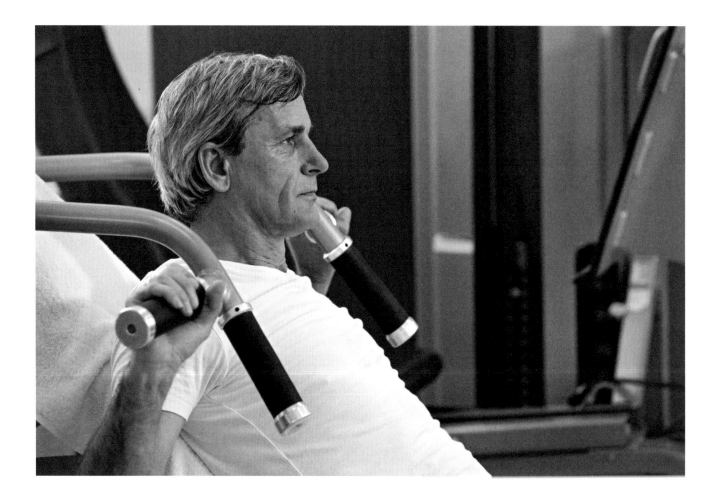

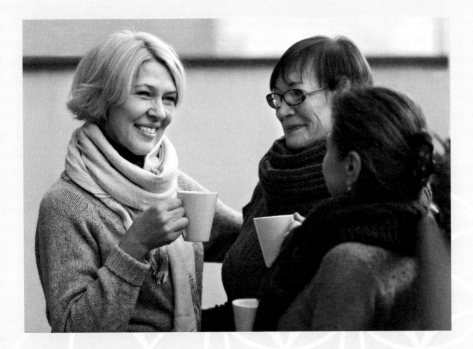

IN PRAISE OF GYM BUDDIES

"You meet the nicest people on a Honda." So went the tagline for one of the most memorable ad campaigns of the 1960s. It popped into my mind the other day when I thought about an updated version: "You meet the nicest people at the dumbbell rack."

Of course, there's no time for socializing when I'm working out with my trainer. He gives me his full attention and expects the same. But I've gotten into the habit of coming in early to warm up, and staying afterward to hit a couple more exercise stations and generally hang out. Otherwise, I would miss connecting with some of the most interesting people I know!

There's the retired botanist, the political junkie, the woman who's written a string of popular novels, the young biochemist who wows me with his handstands, the former Army Ranger who tells amazing stories, the grad student soon to leave for a year in China...a whole group of fascinating folks who work out on a schedule similar to mine. It's like attending the best party ever—without the temptation of drinking and eating too much.

My gym buddies are people I wouldn't ordinarily meet—and they've opened up my world in ways I could never have imagined. We also act as each other's fitness cheerleaders and share things we've learned about working out. Sometimes we even find moments for deep conversation amid the cables and machines.

I'm not the only one who has gained a new social circle and some enduring relationships by being a gym regular. I see clusters of people staying to chat or making plans to meet for lunch. A few of my buddies have become full-fledged friends I invite for a hike or a glass of wine. At a time in my life when I'm out of the workplace, old friends are moving away, and my social connections could be dwindling, my cup runneth over.

JACKIE, 67

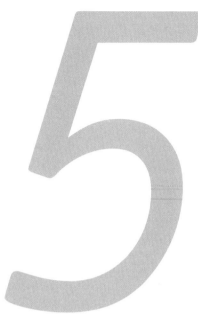

BASIC EXERCISES, *PROGRESSED*

IN THE LAST CHAPTER, I introduced five basic exercises as the starting point for a continuing workout program. I chose them not only because these movements are powerful *and* safe, if done with proper form, but also because all five can be either regressed or progressed. They can be made easier for strength-training newbies, or harder for seasoned workout mavens—which is what you will be if you keep working at it!

What follows are examples of the directions in which you can take the same five classic exercises once you've got the basic versions nailed. This is less about which specific versions you *should* do, and more about offering ideas as to what you *can* do. The variations are almost endless. What I hope you will take away from this chapter is the principle of progression, and an understanding of how much you can gain by taking familiar exercises into new territory.

I can hear the reactions now: are you saying a push-up isn't hard *enough*? That's what I felt, too, when I first started doing them. But as I've learned, there are good reasons to keep classic exercises in your repertoire, but move up to different—and more difficult—versions as you get stronger.

First of all, it's a way to add challenge to exercises without spending more time. Once you've worked at the push-up for a while and can handily do 20 or 25 repetitions, you may find it tedious to shoot for 30, 40, or 50 reps in a set.

Secondly, even small variations in an exercise can change which muscles are engaged. Do a push-up with your feet elevated, and the effort is more focused on your upper chest. Meanwhile, because of the angle, you're getting less help from the triceps muscle of your upper arm. Take the same basic push-up exercise and move your hands closer together. Suddenly you're giving your triceps more of a workout. These variations can be useful if you want to challenge one muscle more than another. There's always something else you can do!

Doing different versions of an exercise can also help you discover which parts of your body aren't quite as strong as others. That's important, because it's often those weak links that make you vulnerable to injury when doing real-life tasks. Varying your routine also helps keep things fresh—no small consideration, if your goal is to keep working out and advancing well into old age.

YES, YOU *CAN* GET OLDER, STRONGER, AND FITTER AT THE SAME TIME.

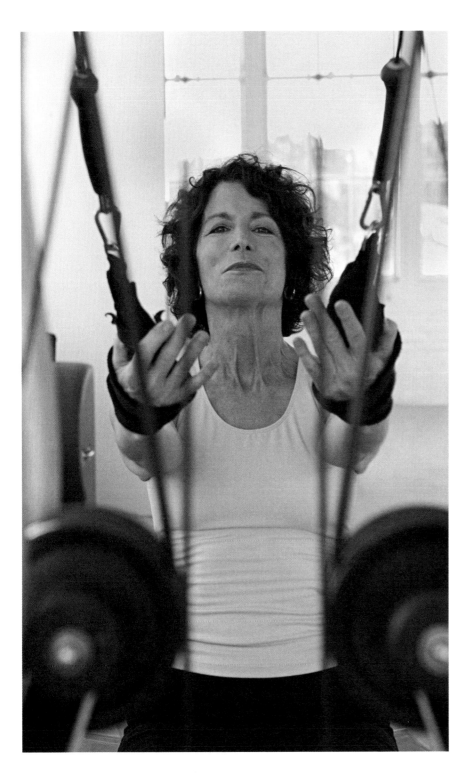

PLANK

BASIC

FORM REMINDERS

- Contract your core muscles throughout.
- Keep your back in a straight line, and don't let your midsection sag.
- Keep breathing!

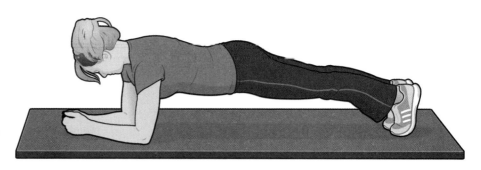

PROGRESSION

SWISS BALL PLANK

You can also use a Bosu or bench to elevate your feet. The higher your feet, the greater the challenge.

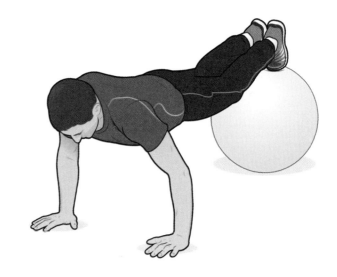

VARIATION

SIDE PLANK

- Lie on one side with your upper body propped up on your forearm and elbow and one foot stacked on the other.
- Make sure your body is in a straight line from ankles to shoulder.
- Try to hold for at least 30 seconds.

Want more challenge?

- Extend your free arm into the air and hold it.
- Try lifting and holding your top leg.

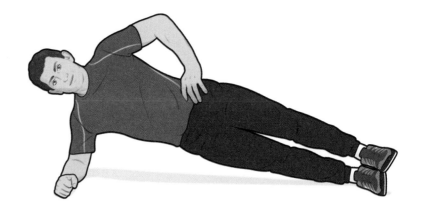

SQUAT

BASIC

FORM REMINDERS

- Keep your sternum lifted.
- Maintain the lumbar curve of your lower back as you make a "sitting" motion.

HARDER

DUMBBELL SQUAT

- Hold a dumbbell in each hand, keeping it in a vertical line as you squat.
- Don't forget—you should always push through your heels as you stand up.
- Start with a light weight and increase gradually.

VARIATION

GOBLET SQUAT (not shown)

- Start with your feet a bit wider than shoulder width with toes pointed slightly outward.
- Using both hands, hold a dumbbell or kettlebell at your chest, keeping it steady as you squat.

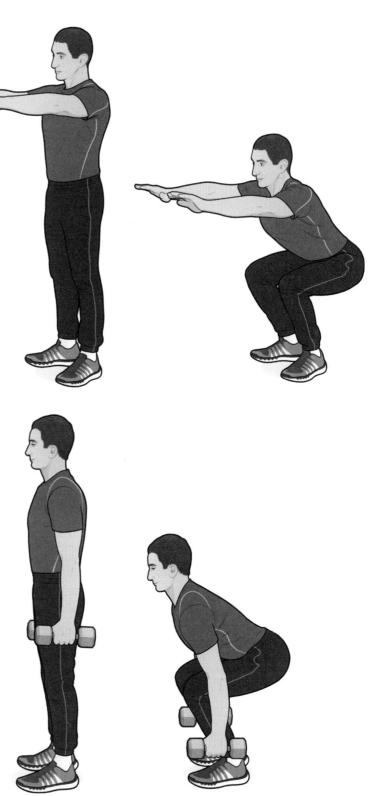

LAT PULLDOWN

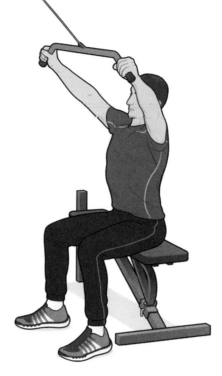
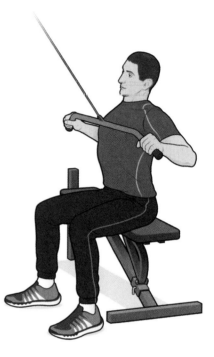

BASIC

FORM REMINDER

- Keep your chest lifted and pull from the lat muscles of your back, not with your hands and arms.

VARIATIONS

1 SINGLE-ARM DUMBBELL ROW

With this version, you are lifting against gravity. It also works one side of your body at a time, so the two sides grow more equal in strength.

- Use your core muscles to keep your back straight as you kneel on the bench.

- Don't look upward; keep your neck in line with your spine.

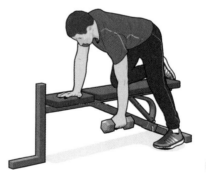
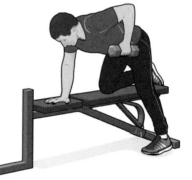

2 INVERTED ROW

- Place your hands at shoulder width or slightly wider.

- Make sure your lats do most of the work, not your arms and shoulders.

Want more challenge?

- Place your feet on a bench so your body is nearly horizontal.

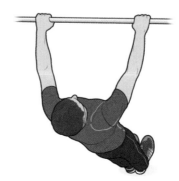
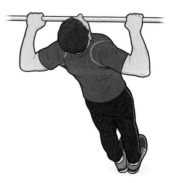

LUNGE

BASIC

FORM REMINDERS

- As you kneel, keep your knee lined up with your ankle and your upper body straight.

- As you stand, push through the heel of your extended leg, not your toes.

HARDER

1 WALKING LUNGE

Find a place in the gym where you can move straight ahead for at least 20 feet.

- Instead of returning to the starting position after a lunge, bring your back foot forward as though you are walking.

- Move forward, repeating with alternating legs.

Want more challenge?

- Do ten steps forward, and ten steps backward.

2 ADD DUMBBELLS

- Increase the challenge to either version by holding dumbbells in each hand.

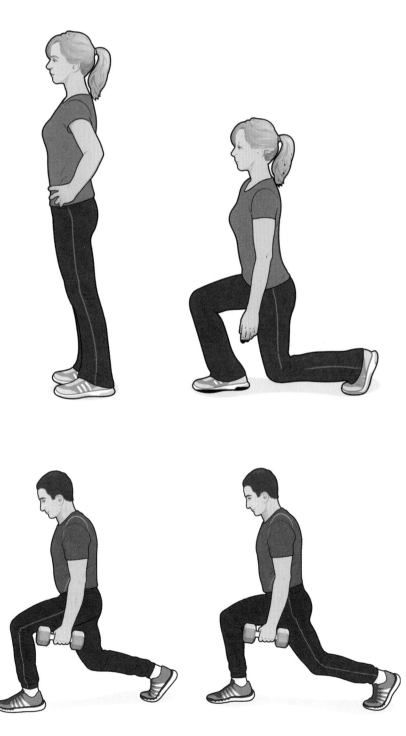

PUSH-UP

BASIC

FORM REMINDERS

- Keep your body in a straight line and your hands about shoulder-width apart.

- Don't let your midsection sag or let gravity take over as you descend.

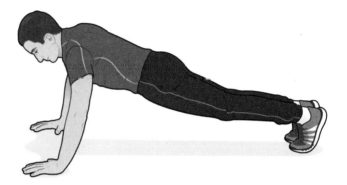

HARDER

DECLINE PUSH-UP

- Elevate your feet on a bench, Swiss ball, or Bosu. The higher your feet, the more the effort will be focused on the upper chest.

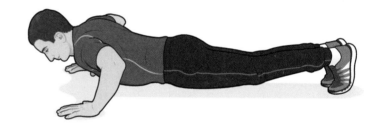

VARIATION

UNSTABLE PUSH-UP

(not shown)

- You can target different muscles by placing your hands on a Swiss ball or a Bosu held with the flat side facing you. The instability adds challenge.

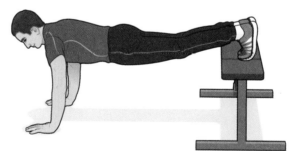

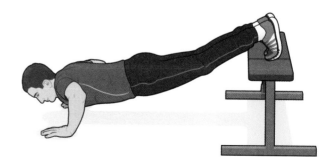

GYM-SPEAK 101

Your body has about 200 skeletal muscles that do most of the work of moving you around. Those labeled here are the major muscles that a full-body workout will typically engage. Once you are working out regularly, you'll soon get to know their names in "gym-speak"—glutes, quads, lats, pecs, and so on. Depending on the physical issues that you and your trainer identify, you may want to give attention to some other smaller or deeper muscles that most classic exercises don't engage.

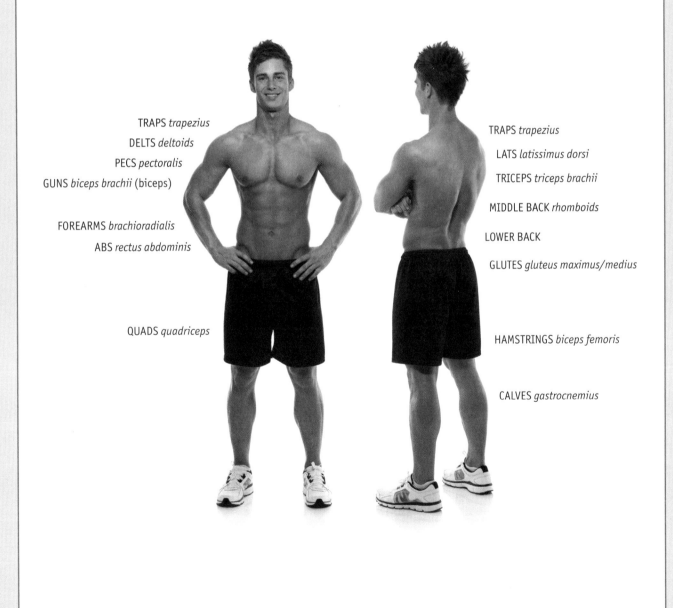

TRAPS *trapezius*
DELTS *deltoids*
PECS *pectoralis*
GUNS *biceps brachii* (biceps)

FOREARMS *brachioradialis*
ABS *rectus abdominis*

QUADS *quadriceps*

TRAPS *trapezius*
LATS *latissimus dorsi*
TRICEPS *triceps brachii*

MIDDLE BACK *rhomboids*

LOWER BACK

GLUTES *gluteus maximus/medius*

HAMSTRINGS *biceps femoris*

CALVES *gastrocnemius*

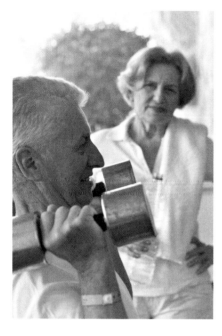

HAVING A PLAN
FOR YOUR WORKOUTS
IS CRITICAL IF YOU
WANT RESULTS.

MAKE SURE YOUR WORKOUT COVERS THE BASES

In order to become functionally fit, you need a full-body workout that will help you build strength in a balanced way. A well designed 60-minute workout should enable you to accomplish that, if you do it consistently and with good effort three times a week. What's more, it will help you improve flexibility and balance at the same time. That's a pretty attractive return for an investment of three hours a week!

Here are my six secrets for structuring a regimen that gets results—things I wish I'd known when I started my fitness journey.

1 DIVIDE YOUR WORKOUT INTO SEGMENTS

This will help you address multiple facets of functional fitness each time you work out. Each 60-minute session should include time specifically allocated to core strength, flexibility, and overall muscular strength.

The graphic in "Anatomy of a Workout" on page 191 is a snapshot of the workout I recommend, based on what has worked for me. Remember that I started as a 70-year-old certified couch potato. If I could do it, odds are you can, too!

The first third of the session is devoted to what you might think of as the opening acts: loosening up with ten minutes of stretching, followed by five minutes of foam rolling, concentrating on areas that are chronically tight, especially hips, glutes, and the hamstring muscles at the back of the thighs. After that comes five minutes for what is labeled "trainer's evaluation" (although it may not take you that long). That's when my trainer and I compare notes on how I'm moving that day and decide on specific exercises to add, vary, or focus on. This helps us adapt our workout to deal with any particular issues that may be cropping up.

From there, it's on to the main event—the day's program of strength-building exercises. In addition to focusing on good form, keep flexibility and balance in mind. You can consciously work to gently extend your range of motion as you do each repetition. You can also include exercises with a balance component, such as movements you do on one leg or on an unstable surface.

Arrive ten minutes before your training appointment so you can warm up on your own. Five minutes on the treadmill, cross-trainer, or stair-climber followed by five minutes of active movement like jumping jacks or seal jacks should get your blood moving.

2 COVER ALL FOUR EXERCISE CATEGORIES

I'm convinced it doesn't really matter which specific exercises you do. What **does** matter is the kinds of exercises you do and how correctly you do them.

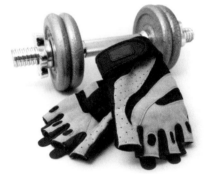

Virtually all strength-building exercises fall into one of four distinct categories. It is no accident that the five classic exercises highlighted in this and the previous chapter cover all four categories, as shown below. To build strength in a balanced way, your workouts should likewise incorporate exercises of all four types. Specifically, I recommend that your routine include:

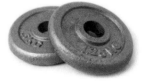

- **Three to four different exercises for core strength.** The plank falls in this category. One set of each should suffice, since the other exercises in your workout will also engage core muscles.

- **Four exercises for overall muscular strength.** Do three sets of 10 to 15 repetitions each. Choose two from the "hip-hinge" category, and one each from the "push" and "pull" categories. I advise doubling down on hip-hinge movements because your lower-body muscles should be the strongest ones in your body. You should be able to accomplish these exercise sets in no more than 30 minutes.

You may want to vary the amount of weight you lift from one set of an exercise to another, especially if you are trying to progress. If so, I recommend that you start light and add weight in the second and/or third sets. While the reverse is common practice, I believe that moving from lighter to heavier weights is a safer approach for folks age 50 and up.

LIFE HAS ITS
UPS AND DOWNS.
WE CALL THEM
"SQUATS."

Please note that the order in which you do the exercises **does** matter. As shown in the graphic, core exercises should always be done first. Because core muscles are the foundation for almost all movements, it only makes sense to activate them early in your session. That way, you'll also avoid fatiguing smaller muscles that you need to support large-muscle movements.

To make your workout more efficient and avoid "overcooking" muscles, do the four overall muscular strength exercises in turn and in this order, one set each: first a hip-hinge, then a push, and then a pull, ending with a different hip-hinge exercise. Repeat this sequence twice, with a brief rest in between, and you're done!

EXAMPLES OF THE FOUR TYPES OF STRENGTH-BUILDING EXERCISES

CORE	HIP-HINGE	PUSH	PULL
Creating tension in your large core muscles	*"Folding" movements with hip & knee flexion*	*Pressing weight away from you*	*Bringing weight toward you*
PLANK	SQUAT / LUNGE	PUSH-UP	LAT PULLDOWN
3 or 4 per session, one set each	2 per session, three sets each	1 per session, three sets each	1 per session, three sets each

3 MOVE IN ALL THREE SPATIAL PLANES

Many exercises involve moving only in the sagittal plane and, for that matter, only in the forward direction. That's also true of walking, running, and bicycling. Your body will be more balanced and stable if you train it to move in all three spatial planes (see page 57). Vary your workout by incorporating some backward, frontal plane (side to side), and transverse plane (rotational) movements at least once over the course of your three weekly workouts. Many exercises have variations that let you move in different planes; the lunge is one of the more versatile examples.

THE THREE SPATIAL PLANES

SAGITTAL	FRONTAL	TRANSVERSE
Forward and backward	*Out to each side*	*In rotation*
LUNGE REVERSE LUNGE	SIDE LUNGE	LUNGE WITH ROTATION

4 EMPHASIZE WHOLE-BODY AND COMPOUND MOVEMENTS

There's nothing inherently wrong with most of the muscle-isolating exercises, such as bicep curls or tricep extensions, that traditional bodybuilders swear by. It may sometimes serve your purpose to focus effort on a single muscle, so long as you don't overdo it. But you will make your workouts more efficient and progress more rapidly if you focus on whole-body movements that engage two or more muscle groups at once. All five of the classic exercises I've recommended fit this criteria.

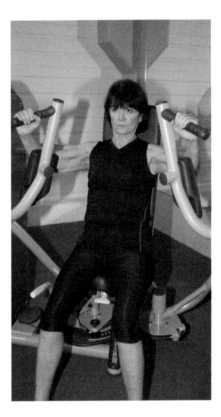

Compound exercises combine what are typically thought of as two different movements. For example, do a squat as you hold two dumbbells at the center of your body, between your legs (keeping your chest up, of course). Then pull the weights toward your shoulders and spiral them upward into a shoulder press as you stand. Compound exercises are closer to the functional movements we do outside the gym. They also add both challenge and efficiency to your workout—a winning combination.

5 TARGET TROUBLE SPOTS

Whether as mainstays or variations in your routine, include some exercises aimed specifically at strengthening your particular areas of vulnerability or weakness, especially those connected with back or joint pain. For example, aching knees might be helped by improving alignment as you walk and move. Similarly, if a shoulder has given you grief in the past, your trainer might suggest ways to strengthen the small muscles of the rotator cuff.

> ### DID YOU KNOW?
>
> *THE HUMAN BODY has between 650 and 840 named skeletal muscles, depending on how you count complex muscles such as the biceps brachii.*

Ask your trainer to focus on causes and remedial strategies rather than simply addressing symptoms. You may want to pull a physical therapist into the discussion if the nature of your problem is unclear. Exercises that get to the root of your issues may be the hardest ones to do well; they're probably also the ones you most need to do.

6 EVOLVE YOUR WORKOUT OVER TIME

You may want to shift the kinds of exercises you do as you progress. When I first began working out, I devoted roughly a third of my training time to core strengthening. While that's more than the average person may require, I sorely needed that focus to help stabilize my chronically bad back. Now that I've got the strong core I was missing, I'm spending more time on exercises to loosen my tight hips and ankles.

You may also want to modify your workout style and activity mix as you get older. Are you noticeably stiffer than you used to be? That may happen even if you stretch, since the body's connective tissue loses water content and becomes less supple with age. Putting more accent on flexibility, and perhaps adding yoga or a tai chi class to your regimen, would be a sensible move. If you notice times when you're unsteady, you should probably increase your training for balance. And if your muscles still feel sore or tired on the third day after a workout, it could be a sign that your body's cellular-level healing processes are slowing down. It may be time to dial back the weight you are lifting and put more focus on ease of movement.

The old cliché about travel also applies to fitness—it's not a destination, but a journey. Like a long trip, it may require different maps at different points. With any luck, it will be an odyssey that lasts the rest of your life.

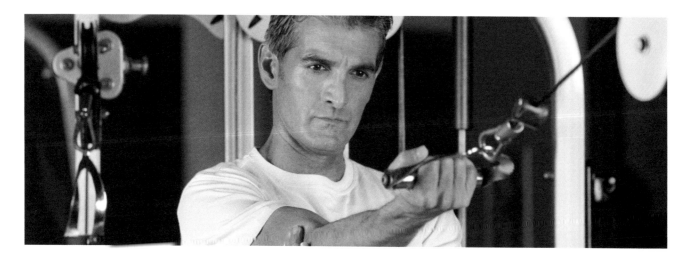

ANATOMY
of a
WORKOUT

MY RECOMMENDED STRUCTURE
FOR A 60-MINUTE WORKOUT

*Be sure to arrive early enough to warm up
on your own before your training appointment.*

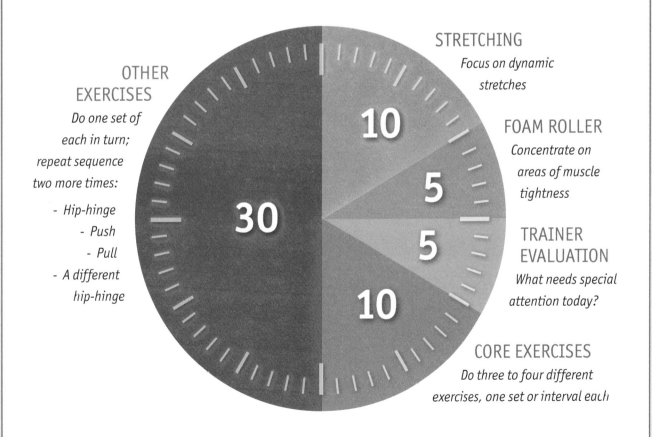

**OTHER
EXERCISES**
*Do one set of
each in turn;
repeat sequence
two more times:*

*- Hip-hinge
- Push
- Pull
- A different
hip-hinge*

30

STRETCHING
*Focus on dynamic
stretches*

10

FOAM ROLLER
*Concentrate on
areas of muscle
tightness*

5

5

**TRAINER
EVALUATION**
*What needs special
attention today?*

10

CORE EXERCISES
*Do three to four different
exercises, one set or interval each*

Common-sense Caveats

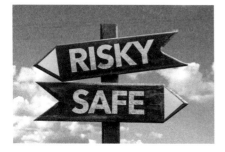

You don't have to be a fitness expert to work out safely. Paying attention to form, staying focused, and listening to your body will go a long way. Here are a few more things you might want to keep in mind.

Progress comes faster on some things than others. With some exercises, I've quickly vaulted ahead. On others, my progress has been slowed by areas of stubborn muscle tightness or lack of joint mobility. But that's how it is for most people. Don't let impatience push you to advance an exercise before your body is ready.

Some exercise machines are safer than others. For example, I'd recommend staying away from leg extension machines that target your quads by having you raise a weight held above your ankles. That is what's called an "open-chain" movement because the body part being exercised moves freely. (A bicep curl is another example.) With those kinds of exercises, the weight is usually far from the center of the body, which increases the stress on joints.

If you're going to use machines, you're better off with the ones designed for "closed-chain" movements, meaning your feet or hands are in a fixed position as you move. Machines like that are generally safer because they compress, stabilize, and help strengthen the joint that is moving.

How much weight you should be lifting isn't always obvious. It's about finding the right balance. Try to lift more than you can handle, and you could suffer a strain or injury that really sets you back. But if you reach for the same very light dumbbells month after month, you won't get any stronger. The ideal weight is just heavy enough to challenge your muscles—and if you're training consistently, that amount will gradually increase over time, until you have reached your goals for strength or hit a natural plateau. Remember that elbows and wrists may not be able to handle as big a load as larger muscles. That's one reason why alignment is so important. The point is, it makes sense to gauge the amount of weight you lift to the weakest link in a chain of movement.

Certain exercises should be off the table. Some moves are inherently risky because they have such a small margin for error; you can hurt yourself with one false move or two seconds of distraction. That's why I would never attempt any exercise that calls for holding or lifting a heavy bar behind my neck. As for kettlebells, I like working out with them, but I'm cautious about it. Kettlebell movements typically involve momentum, and you don't want to let it take you places your body isn't prepared to go.

Beyond that, you may have a past injury or some other physical condition that limits what you can do. If so, talk with your trainer (and perhaps your doctor or physical therapist) about any kinds of exercises you should modify or avoid altogether. In any case, don't ever be shy about telling a trainer, "I'm afraid I might hurt myself if I do that." Any good trainer will suggest an equally effective alternative.

Pain signals should never be ignored. I'm not talking about the muscle soreness you get after a strenuous workout, which generally fades after two or three days. By "pain," I mean the kind of hurt that tells you something is amiss, whether due to a wrong move or a chronic injury. Anytime you feel a painful pull, "tweak," sprain, or strain—whether during your workout or some other physical activity—immediately stop what you're doing.

Don't ever "work through" the pain. If you can't move the injured part or put any weight on it, see your doctor or go to the emergency room right away. Otherwise, use the standard RICE treatment: rest, ice, compression, and elevation of the injured part.

Chronic injuries call for an action plan. If you have a chronic or lingering injury, it makes sense to see your doctor and develop a rehabilitation plan with help from your trainer and physical therapist. They may recommend work-arounds (such as lighter weights or alternative movements) so you can keep up your conditioning while you heal as well as exercises to strengthen supporting muscles. Be patient as your body heals—it may take weeks or, in some cases, even months—but be proactive, too. Don't resign yourself to a physical limitation if you haven't actively worked to restore full functioning.

Safety comes first. Don't ever try a new exercise or piece of workout equipment without being shown the correct form. Also, when learning a new movement, be sure to start with minimal weight or body weight alone, increasing it only in small increments and only when you are confident of your form. Err on the side of caution whenever you are in doubt.

Prevention is the best policy. Getting stronger will help you avoid hurting yourself, especially if you strengthen muscle groups that support and stabilize injury-prone areas of the body such as legs, ankles, knees, shoulders, and the lower back. You can also prevent injuries by warming up before you work out, cross-training with a variety of physical activities that engage different muscle groups, and giving your body enough time to rest between workouts.

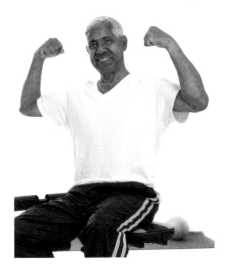

GETTING RESULTS
YOU CAN SEE AND
FEEL IS THE BEST
MOTIVATOR OF ALL.

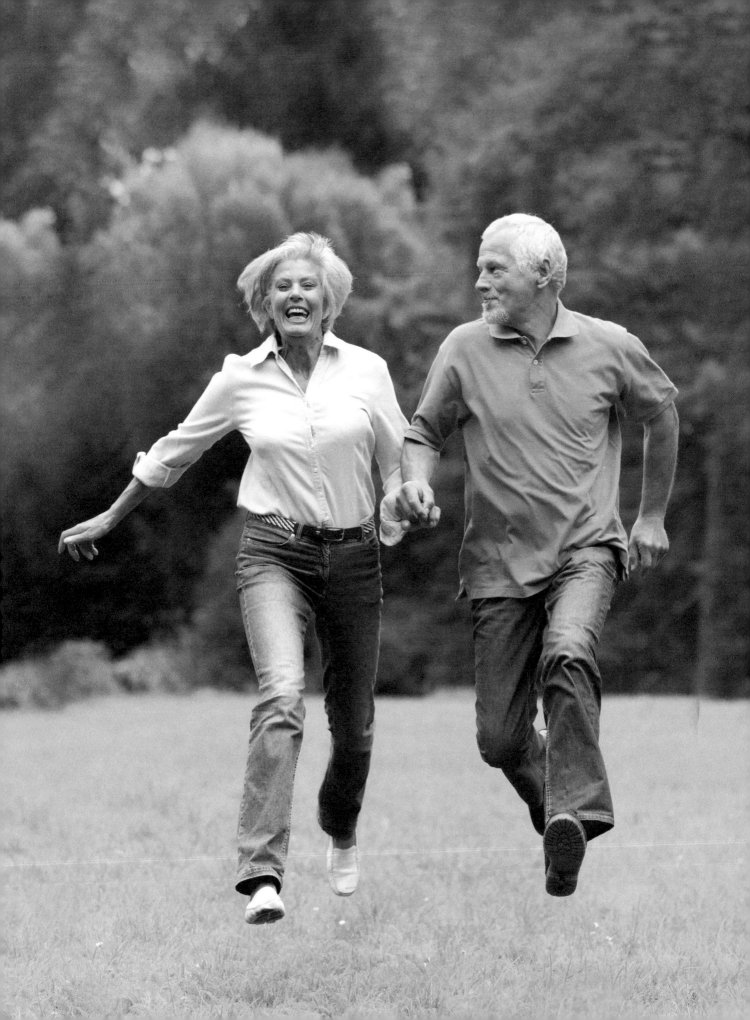

CHAPTER NINE

A Few Closing Thoughts
It's All About You

THERE'S A GOOD REASON why this book is titled *Just Move!*, and I want to circle back to it before you take in these last few pages. I hope my central message comes through loud and clear: **doing something** to preserve and improve your functional fitness is absolutely essential if you care about your quality of life as you age. Some people are 60 years old, but look and feel like 80. Others are 80, but look and feel more like 60—and wouldn't we all rather be in that group?

What I've shared in these pages is my approach to lifelong fitness, based on what has worked for me. But the only thing that matters is what works for you. Exercise is something you do for yourself, and a program can succeed only if it is embraced by you, customized for you, and becomes part of your life.

This is why I would never say that you "should" follow what I've done or "must" advance through all four steps. There is no one fitness template that works for everyone. Nor is there any moral rectitude in being able to touch your toes or do a perfect push-up. There is no point in focusing on what you can't do or don't want to do.

Focus on what you *can* do, and go from there. Keep it positive, and concentrate on the physical activities you enjoy and, thus, are more apt to stick with. In short, it's all good, as long as you **just move.** In that spirit, here are a few last thoughts on mapping your own fitness journey.

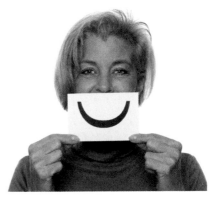

NO ONE FITNESS TEMPLATE WORKS FOR EVERYONE. WHAT MATTERS IS WHAT WORKS FOR *YOU*.

THE "RIGHT" FITNESS PROGRAM IS THE ONE THAT FITS YOUR GOALS

Some people are hard chargers who like to test themselves and enjoy physical challenges. Others don't want to work that hard; they simply want to look and feel a little better. If that describes you, you may decide that a simple program of regular stretching and walking suits your needs just fine. If you can eventually add some basic exercises, a movement class, or a sport you enjoy, so much the better.

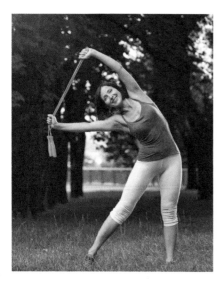

WHAT IF A GYM AND TRAINER AREN'T POSSIBLE?

Maybe you live far from any good gym, or don't want to spend money on a trainer, or can't be tied into scheduled appointments. If so, not to worry. Those circumstances need not stand in the way of getting fit. While it's advantageous to have a trainer and work out in a gym, there are certainly other ways you can go.

If there are no well-equipped gyms near you, you may find alternatives at your local community center, Y, medical center, hospital, high school, or college. You could even check out nearby hotels, which will often let area residents use their gyms and pools for a small fee. And don't forget the great outdoors! Some parks have parcourses that feature jogging or walking trails punctuated by exercise stations; playgrounds may also provide equipment you can use or adapt for certain exercises.

Of course, there is also the option of working out at home. You'll notice that four of the five basic exercises highlighted in Chapters 7 and 8 rely on body weight and can be done virtually anywhere. As for the fifth, the lat pulldown, you can easily put together a substitute for that machine with a set of elastic resistance bands and a pull-up bar that fits any standard doorway. Both items can be found online or at a sporting goods store for less than $50.

When you don't have a trainer, it's up to you to be a good student of exercise form. But those are principles you need to be learning, anyway. You can do it on your own if you take the tips in Chapter 7 to heart, pay close attention as you exercise, and take things one step at a time.

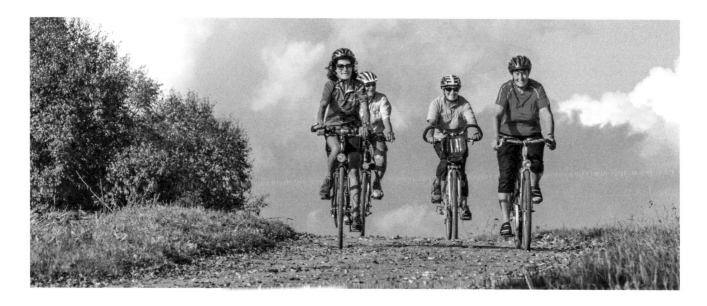

IT GETS EASIER AS YOU PROGRESS

Once you've got the fitness habit, and some grasp of good form and technique, you can expect to see tangible results. In my experience, that is the best motivator of all. It took me three years of consistent workouts and steady improvement to reach the point of being truly fit. It may take you more or less time.

Then you're in the realm of staying fit—and that's a lot more fun. By then you've learned how to work out efficiently. You've got the confidence to try new things. And you can keep selectively raising the bar, if you want. One thing I've added to my workouts is 60-second intervals of fast-paced, anaerobic exercises such as jumping jacks. Doing one minute of conditioning at three points during my strength workout has made a big difference in my stamina and helped me get leaner.

Or, if you prefer, you can switch into maintenance mode on strength training and spend more time on other physical activities you enjoy. However you mix things up, you can stay fit if you keep up the basic discipline: an hour a day, six days a week.

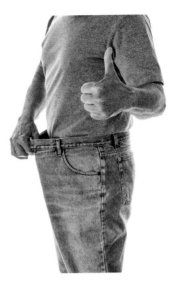

YOU CAN DO IT!
JUST KEEP MAKING
GOOD CHOICES,
ONE DAY AT A TIME.

EXTRA POUNDS CAN BE A HINDRANCE

I'm not talking about having a full-figured body type or a couple of bulges you'd rather not see in the mirror. But if you've got too much excess weight, it can significantly increase your cardiovascular load, put more pressure on joints, and accelerate the loss of cartilage, especially when it comes to weight-bearing joints such as knees and hips. Every 10 pounds of excess weight around your middle exerts 40 pounds of added pressure on the knees, according to Dr. Eric Matteson, chair of the Mayo Clinic's rheumatology division.

If weight is an issue, it's probably a good idea to accompany your new workout routine with a nutritional makeover. One program will reinforce the other, and you'll look and feel better that much faster.

Before you embark on a weight-loss program, however, it's a good idea to do some research. When *U.S. News & World Report* asked a panel of health experts to rate the safety and effectiveness of weight-loss diets, they chose the DASH diet, a relatively obscure program originally developed to fight high blood pressure, as the best all-around approach. Their top ten list includes popular commercial diets that provide hand-holding and support as well as do-it-yourself regimens developed by the National Institutes of Health and the Mayo Clinic. Personally, I follow a modified Mediterranean diet, but different diets work for different people.

DON'T EAT
ANYTHING YOUR
GREAT-GRANDMOTHER
WOULDN'T RECOGNIZE
AS FOOD.

MICHAEL POLLAN
Food Rules

CALORIES COUNT, EVEN WHEN YOU'RE WORKING OUT

"Abs are made in the kitchen," goes a saying common in fitness circles. It's a shorthand way of saying that what you eat has a great deal more impact on your weight than what you do for exercise. It may take several hours of intensive cardiovascular activity to burn off the calories in that slice of cheesecake or bag of chips. So don't let an eating binge after your workout undo its caloric-torching benefits.

The good news is that exercise doesn't make you hungrier, researchers say. In fact, it may actually blunt your appetite by lowering your body's level of ghrelin, the hormone that stimulates hunger. Cardio exercise, in particular, also increases levels of a hunger-suppressing hormone, peptide YY. If you feel ravenous after a workout, that may be a matter of habit or wanting a reward. It could also be because your last meal was hours earlier. Having a banana, a handful of almonds, or some Greek yogurt an hour before your session should help you avoid hunger pangs during or right after your workout. I also find that a small cup of black coffee a half hour before my workout gives me a boost and keeps my appetite in check.

TOO MUCH SITTING CAN UNDERMINE YOUR EFFORTS

All the stretching in the world won't help you stay flexible if you can't break the habit of sitting. There's also the fact that sitting is strongly correlated with elevated risks of serious disease and premature death. Research suggests that the critical factor may not be the total amount of time you sit; it's the number of hours spent sitting immobile (see page 26). So think about strategies for

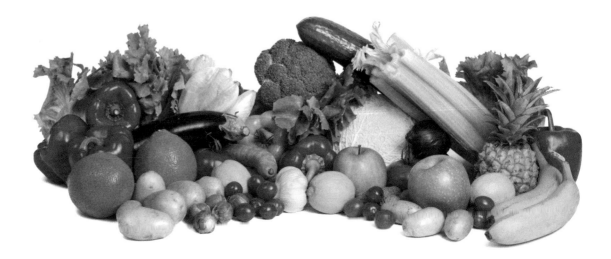

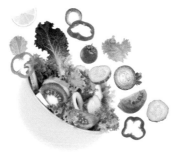

IF YOU WANT TO BE ACTIVE and build lean muscle, your body needs the right fuel. But good nutrition doesn't have to be complicated or boring. It's mainly a matter of eating "leaner and cleaner." Your waistline and your workouts will benefit, and your taste buds may like it, too. Food tastes better when the natural flavors of good ingredients shine through. Despite all the food fads and controversies out there, medical experts generally agree on the basics of good nutrition:

Eat a variety of nutrient-dense foods, including enough high-quality protein (see pages 76–77), plenty of fruits and vegetables, and a moderate amount of "good" carbohydrates, such as whole grains and sweet potatoes.

Limit sugar and sodium. This is important for managing your weight, but also for reducing risk factors for heart disease, stroke, and diabetes. Getting in the habit of reading food labels helps. Look at sodium content, for example, and you'll find that much of what we consume doesn't come from the salt shaker but is hidden in processed foods like bread or salad dressing.

Eat based on hunger, not the clock. The old idea of eating "three squares a day" can lead to eating more than we need. It also causes us to eat out of habit or in response to external cues rather than genuine hunger. Pay attention to your body's hunger signals, and you should be able to find the pattern of meals and small snacks that works best for you. Just be sure to stop eating when you're full, and snack only when you truly need a boost.

Practice portion control. Serve food on smaller plates; research shows that eating from large plates makes us think we're eating less than we really are. Follow the Japanese principle of *hara hachi bu,* which means "eat until you are 80 percent full." It helps if you eat slowly; it takes about 20 minutes for your digestive system to register what you've eaten, and you'll feel more satisfied if you savor each mouthful. When eating out, choose from the small plates, appetizers, and salads, or split an entrée with your companion.

Choose "real food" over processed "food products," which are often high in sugar, sodium, and chemical additives, and low in nutritional quality. As author Michael Pollan puts it in his book *Food Rules:* "Don't eat anything your great-grandmother wouldn't recognize as food" (though tofu might be one exception).

Pay attention to ingredients and preparation methods. Cross anything fried off your list, and remember that salads aren't always low-cal—not when they are loaded with dressing, bacon, or cheese. Many restaurant salads weigh in at well over 1,000 calories.

Stay away from fad diets and "miracle" ingredients. The secret to losing pounds and managing your weight is no secret at all: limit calories, eat the right foods, and get regular exercise. If you have always struggled with your weight or need to lose a significant amount, you may want to consider consulting a bariatric physician.

Make smart swaps, like substituting mustard or yogurt for mayonnaise, chicken or turkey for beef, a side of sliced tomatoes or fruit in place of French fries. Shaving just 250 or so calories a day will add up to a two-pound weight loss over the course of a month. That's not so hard to do. When it comes to managing your weight, it's the accretion of small choices you make each day that will determine your long-run success.

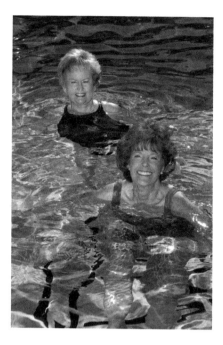

FIND WAYS TO MOVE
THAT YOU ENJOY.

cutting down on extended chair time. If you use a cell phone, you can be up and moving around as you talk. And if you're reading, working, or watching TV, don't let more than 20 or 30 minutes go by without getting up for a stretch or a drink of water. Here again, "just move" is the watchword.

EARNING RESPECT IN THE GYM ISN'T DIFFICULT

It's not a matter of how much weight you can lift or how many repetitions you can do. Trust me, nobody cares about that. What your trainer and fellow gym patrons will notice is the intensity of your focus, the quality of your exercise form, and the level of effort you put into your workout. Those are the things that win admiration, and they are all within your control.

LOVE YOURSELF, LOVE YOUR WORKOUT

We all know fitness is important if we want to stay active and energetic in our later years. So why do so many people have a hard time getting into and sticking with a training program?

Research tells us that extrinsic motivations—long-term, future-oriented rewards like lowering blood pressure or looking good at a class reunion— don't have much staying power. If you exercise because your doctor or spouse says you must, it turns your workouts into an obligation and a chore.

Far more effective are intrinsic motivators—the kind that come from within— especially if they concern your current state of being. Studies show that people who enjoy physical training and think of it as a way to feel good are far more likely to exercise regularly. Finding some kind of movement you truly enjoy makes a big difference, because it connects exercise with feelings of pleasure. I know one woman who finds exhilaration in "solo dance parties" that involve nothing more than moving to favorite playlists with no one else around. It also helps if you associate workouts with good things like having time to yourself, making social connections, or accomplishing what you set out to do.

Best of all, researchers say, is a blend of intrinsic and extrinsic motivators strongly reinforced by habit and a positive attitude. So think of your fitness program as something you do for yourself and, while you're at it, for those who love you and want you to enjoy your life for many years to come.

THE ULTIMATE REWARD

WORKING OUT IS FUN? "C'mon Jim...you can't be serious." I've grown accustomed to hearing incredulous comments like that from my friends and associates.

I just smile. I've learned there is plenty of fun to be found in getting and staying fit, and I hope this book well help you discover that for yourself.

It's fun to feel—I mean *really feel*—the sensations of your body in action, especially if you haven't paid much attention to it in years. I almost never fail to leave a workout session feeling happier, more energetic, and more upbeat than when I arrived.

It's fun to take on a physical challenge you could never have managed before, and enjoy that burst of pride when you succeed. It's also fun to learn new things, especially when you're older and supposedly in your dotage. The kinetic chain...the right ways and wrong ways to move...the magic of standing up straight and breathing properly...these are all things I never knew before, and I'm profiting immensely from knowing them now.

Seeing yourself getting visibly stronger, leaner, and more flexible? That's fun, too, and it only whets the appetite for new accomplishments. Success breeds success. We all know it's fun to be a winner, and that's what you are whenever you achieve a personal best.

What people often overlook, however, is how becoming physically fit can bring deep feelings of satisfaction—even joy—to the later chapters of life.

When you are functionally fit, and can go through your day with relative ease, you feel more at home in your own skin. The pleasures of moving also take the sting from the inevitable outward signs of age. Self-acceptance and serenity are closer at hand.

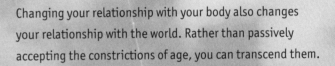

Changing your relationship with your body also changes your relationship with the world. Rather than passively accepting the constrictions of age, you can transcend them.

You don't have to say no to experiences just because you're not mobile or energetic enough to partake of them. You can choose to say yes to life, and be open to all the richness and wonder the world has to offer.

Aches, pains, and stiffness are reminders that your body is built to move, regardless of age. Respond with any kind of movement you enjoy, and it will thank you. Choose the path of fitness, and your body will repay you. You will feel and be more fully *alive*—and isn't that the best reward of all?

JIM OWEN

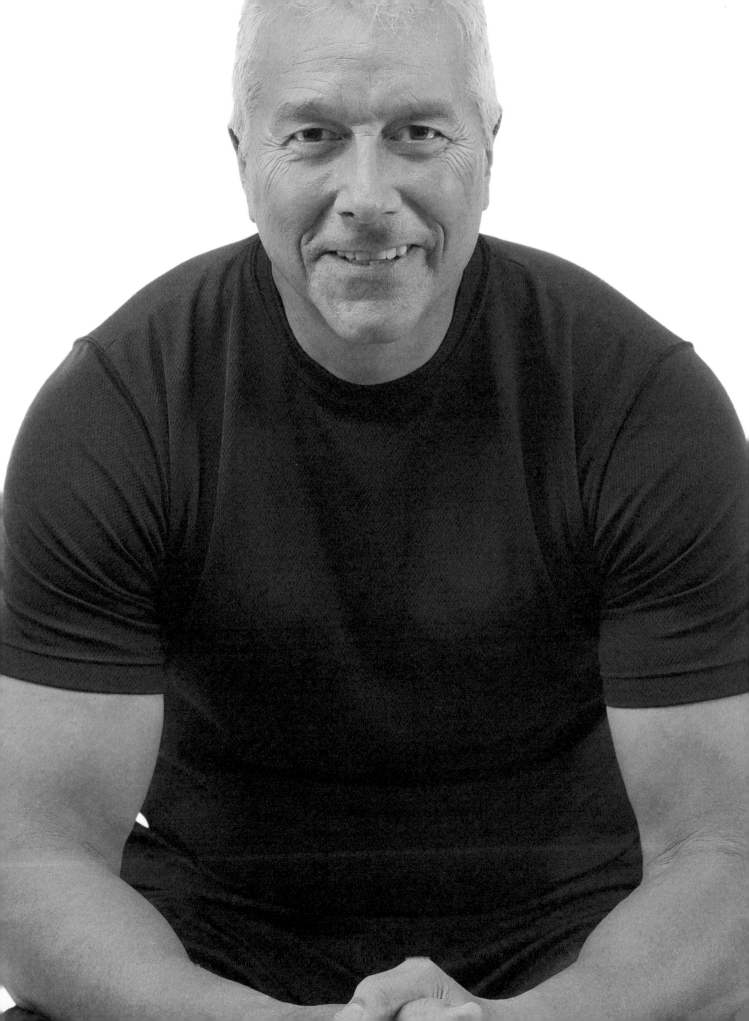

TEN TAKEAWAYS

1 YOU HAVE MORE CONTROL OVER THE AGING PROCESS THAN YOU THINK.

2 WHAT MATTERS AFTER 50 IS FUNCTIONAL FITNESS— BEING ABLE TO HANDLE LIFE'S DAILY PHYSICAL DEMANDS.

4 TO SUCCEED AT FITNESS, YOU NEED TO MAKE IT A WAY OF LIFE.

3 FUNCTIONAL FITNESS HAS FIVE DIMENSIONS; CARDIO ALONE ISN'T ENOUGH.

5 START WITH WHAT YOU CAN DO, AND MAKE SMALL, STEADY IMPROVEMENTS FROM THERE.

6 YOU CAN GET FIT IF YOU WORK AT IT FOR ONE HOUR A DAY, SIX DAYS A WEEK.

7 LEARNING TO STAND STRAIGHT AND BREATHE DEEPLY WILL START YOU ON THE ROAD TO SUCCESS.

8 THE QUALITY OF YOUR FOCUS, EFFORT, AND ATTENTION TO FORM WILL DETERMINE YOUR RESULTS.

9 WHAT YOU DO OUTSIDE THE GYM MATTERS AS MUCH AS YOUR WORKOUT.

10 JUST MOVE! AND DON'T FORGET TO HAVE FUN DOING IT!

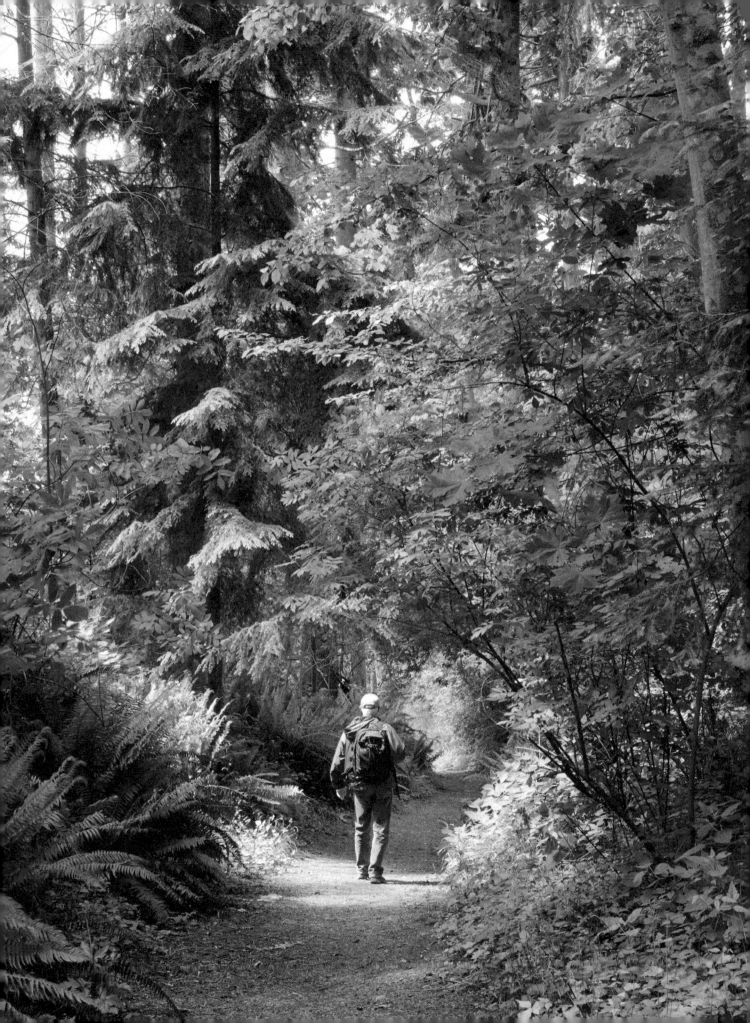

The Journey Continues
Who's Who in Functional Fitness

I invite you to follow me as I connect with top trainers, physical therapists, and other fitness experts around the country. What's different about getting fit after 50? How is the movement toward functional fitness evolving? What lessons and inspiration can we gain from the many success stories out there? Let's explore the fitness landscape together.

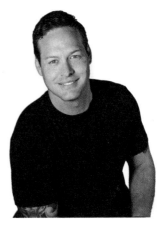

THE FIRST STOP on my continuing education tour: the Four Seasons Resort at Las Colinas in Dallas, Texas. There I was lucky to snag a workout with Josh Biard, who directs all fitness activities at the resort's Sports Club. As I soon discovered, the Las Colinas resort is like an amusement park for people who love to be physically active.

What intrigued me most was the new functional fitness studio recently added as part of an $8 million, two-year renovation. That's where I worked out with Josh, who gave me some new twists on classic exercises along with plenty of food for thought.

JOSH BIARD
Athletic Performance Manager
THE SPORTS CLUB, FOUR SEASONS RESORT
AT LAS COLINAS
Dallas, Texas

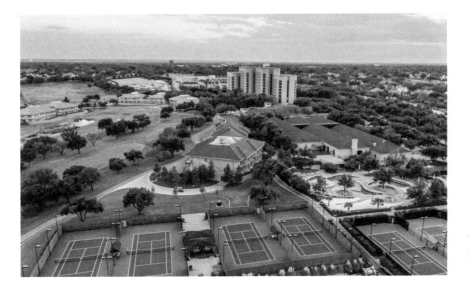

visit us at
justmoveforlife.com

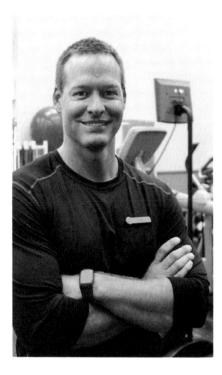

Growing up in Telluride, Colorado, I was always into skiing, snowboarding, and other kinds of sports. I got my personal training certification so I could work part-time while studying at Arizona State University. At first I had no intention of making it a career, but I soon realized I had a passion for it. By the time I was 20, I had started my own training business. Eventually I built three personal training businesses in Colorado, Kentucky, and Arizona, where I worked with a lot of NFL players.

Having done my own thing, I never thought I would be working for a company like the Four Seasons. But this is a unique property, and I saw the opportunity to help build something special here. I'm in charge of the whole fitness side of the resort, including a staff of 11 personal trainers. We have all the components of fitness—a PGA golf course, tennis courts, an indoor running track, squash courts, a rock-climbing wall, 176,000 square feet of fitness equipment and facilities—just about everything you could imagine.

There's a scientific approach to wellness here. As far as I know, we're the only place in Dallas that does Bod Pod testing, which uses air compression to quickly and accurately analyze your body's proportions of fat and lean muscle. We build nutritional programs for people based in part on their VO_2, an indicator of the rate at which they burn calories when at rest. We help them figure out what kinds of exercise to do, calculate their ideal walking rate, and work with them to come up with a complete program.

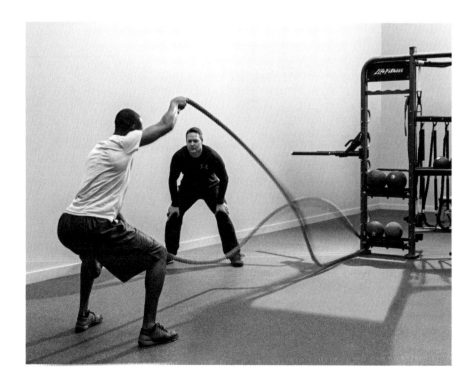

This club is also unique in having an entire studio devoted to functional training. That's a different training concept because it moves away from the machines and muscle-isolating exercises many people are accustomed to. It centers instead on the kinds of functional movements you use in your life. My philosophy is that every workout should use every single muscle group. That kind of training conditions your body and your mind so you can comfortably do things like bend down and pick something up. You can do that movement in the right way, the way you did it in the gym, without having to think about it.

People in our country today really suffer from living sedentary, desk- and chair-bound lives. I've studied ancestral health, and even though people had shorter life spans generations ago, they had less illness and better bone density because they were in constant motion. My grandfather, who is 88, has a logging company in Telluride. He still logs every day and is in phenomenal shape!

That way of life isn't possible for most people, but functional training is the next best thing. In my experience, it's the quickest and most effective way to offset a sedentary lifestyle. That's why I recommend it for people of any age, especially those over 50, because it promotes quality of life, helps you accomplish daily activities, and prevents injuries as you get older. It has nothing to do with bulking up. It's all about feeling good and helping you function in your life. As a side effect, you'll look good, too.

OLDER PEOPLE UNDERESTIMATE WHAT THEY CAN DO.

ONCE THEY HAVE THE RIGHT FOUNDATION, THEY CAN PROGRESS FASTER THAN THEY EVER IMAGINED.

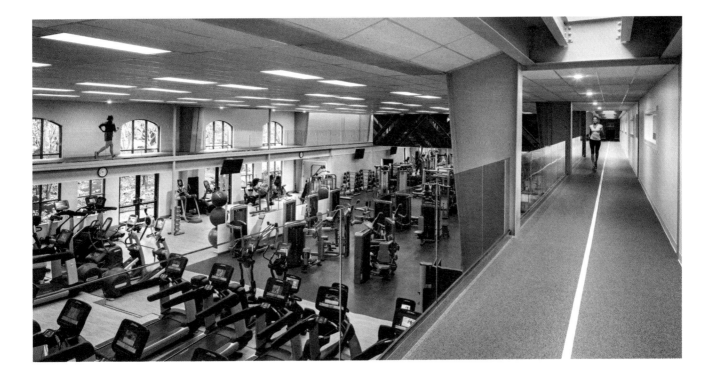

I'VE NEVER ENCOUNTERED SOMEONE TOO OLD FOR SOME KIND OF PHYSICAL ACTIVITY.

Many trainers have concerns about working with older people because it takes more time to lay the groundwork. They also worry that clients might get injured. Most older people have had years of being sedentary or training the wrong way, so they have muscle imbalances. If they've worked out at all, they've usually stayed with the treadmill or bike, or done circuit training with muscle-isolating machines.

With clients over 50, our approach is to start slow and progress at a measured pace. You have to build the foundation of core strength before you can do anything requiring a lot of balance or movement of joints. That's why working with older people is different. Often you have to start from the ground up. Moving with correct form is critical, but you have to be capable of doing that. Someone who's over 50 or 60 may not have the strength or control to do a proper squat at the outset. But once they start getting stronger and improving their balance, they can progress just as quickly as someone who's 30.

At the beginning, our workouts are an hour long, because you need that time to focus on basics and work on details. After we've worked together for a while, they typically evolve to 45- and then 30-minute sessions. We pick up the pace and streamline everything so you're working smarter, not harder, as you get in better shape. By then, you're able to do five times more exercise in 30 minutes than you were doing before in an hour. What's more, you can do it without worries about getting hurt. If you're doing functional training the right way, with a focus on whole-body and multimovement exercises that mimic how your body moves naturally, you're eliminating the muscular imbalances that cause injuries in the first place.

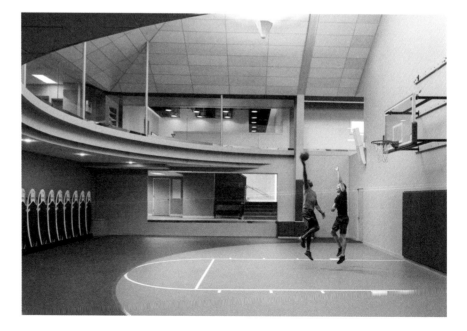

The biggest challenge for most older people is getting over the initial hump. They're afraid they won't be able to do it or have a fear of getting hurt. Those who have been mostly sedentary, or are used to machines where they're moving in just one plane, may find functional training a little scary at first. That's why having a trainer who understands that approach is important. When you're stepping out of your comfort zone, you need someone to guide you. That's especially important if you need to adapt your program for conditions like arthritis. It might be a slower progression, but you'll still get there—and you'll feel so much better when you're doing the right exercises.

Most of the time, older clients are surprised by what they can do and how fast they progress. They go from "I can't get up the stairs" to "Hey, now I'm jogging up the stairs!" Their pains may disappear, even when their doctors have told them they will suffer pain for the rest of their life. With the right exercises and right techniques, there is something they can do. They really can turn back the clock. I've got a client in his fifties whom I'd put up against any 22-year-old. I have also trained people who were in their nineties. I've never encountered anyone too old for some kind of physical activity.

Once a client is up to speed with a program of functional exercise at least two or three times a week, we keep setting new goals. Continuing to progress and improve is extremely important. Without that, you're going to hit a wall and begin to devolve, so you develop muscular imbalances and increase your chances of injury. Remember that progress doesn't necessarily mean doing more; it means getting more efficient so you're doing the same work or more in less time.

Mixing things up is equally important. Your body will do better with more variety. Here at our club, we have 60 different group exercise classes along with all the other activities. You've got to be intelligent about it, and give your body a day to recover from a full-body day. But I love to hear that in between, my clients are doing yoga, going to a barre class or a swim class—the more, the better. Go out and walk or hike on varied terrain. Do things you're not doing in your workout.

The fun comes in having new challenges and accomplishments. I find my clients enjoy things like time challenges, where you're trying to beat the clock as you do a certain amount. Then you train for three more weeks and try it again. It's a real boost when you achieve a new personal best. We also use some fun stuff like a bar with weighted ends that looks like a medieval mace. In functional training a lot of the movements are fun, too. Doing one-legged squats or rotations with the TRX straps gives your workout a different dimension. You're not going up against anyone else. It's all about you.

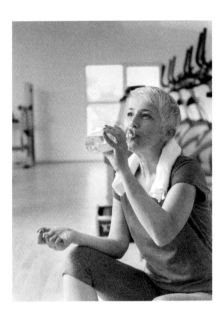

IT'S A REAL BOOST WHEN YOU ACHIEVE A NEW PERSONAL BEST.

The Workout

Focus
Form
Effort

"INTENSE" is a good word to describe the hour I spent working out with Josh Biard in the Four Seasons functional fitness studio. I told him I wanted to be tested, and he certainly delivered! Josh's workout called for my best focus, form, and effort, and I gave it everything I had.

As it turned out, our progression of exercises mapped neatly to the template I normally use, incorporating core, hip-hinge, push, and pull movements. Still, the workout was far from predictable, and Josh took several familiar exercises to a whole new level. It was definitely fun to work out in the studio, which is furnished mainly for bodyweight exercises rather than being cluttered with the usual thicket of machines.

For me, the biggest fun factor was Josh himself. He kept things moving, offered great pointers on form, and threw in a few surprises to boot. I hope to get a spot on his calendar next time I'm in Dallas.

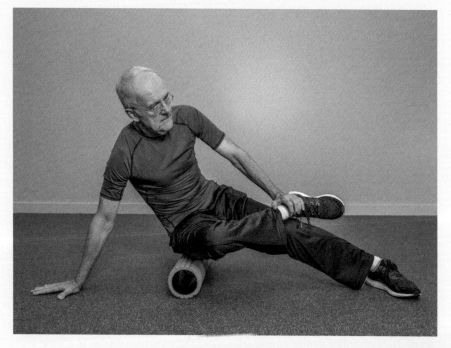

WARM-UP
Like me, Josh is a big believer in warm-ups that include foam rolling to loosen areas of tightness.

ALL PHOTOS BY JIM HAVEY, HAVEY PRODUCTIONS

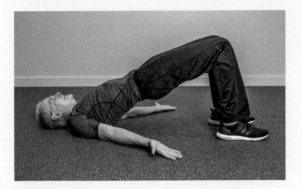

BRIDGE

If you've got tight hips like me, the bridge is a must-do. It's a stretch I always enjoy in my warm-up.

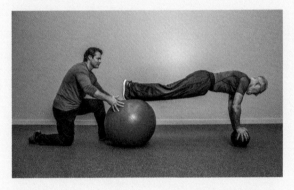

PLANK

This core movement is a basic, but Josh adds a challenging progression. The fun begins when he lets go of the ball—and you're on your own!

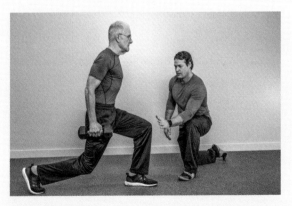

LUNGE

Josh teaches good form with tried-and-true exercises like this one. Here he reminds me to keep my knee from going past my toes.

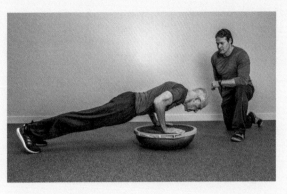

PUSH-UP

The instability of doing push-ups with a Bosu makes it harder to hold the ideal straight-arrow back position.

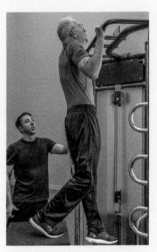

WIDE-GRIP PULL-UP

These are tough no matter how you cut it. Josh's assistant, Matt Greenemeier, guides me to pull more from the lat muscles of my back, and less from my biceps and shoulders.

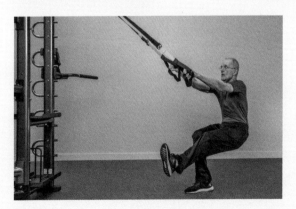

ONE-LEGGED SQUAT

New for me, but Josh assured me I could do it safely by using the TRX straps for stability. I glowed with pride when he complimented my form—a great way to wind up an altogether satisfying workout.

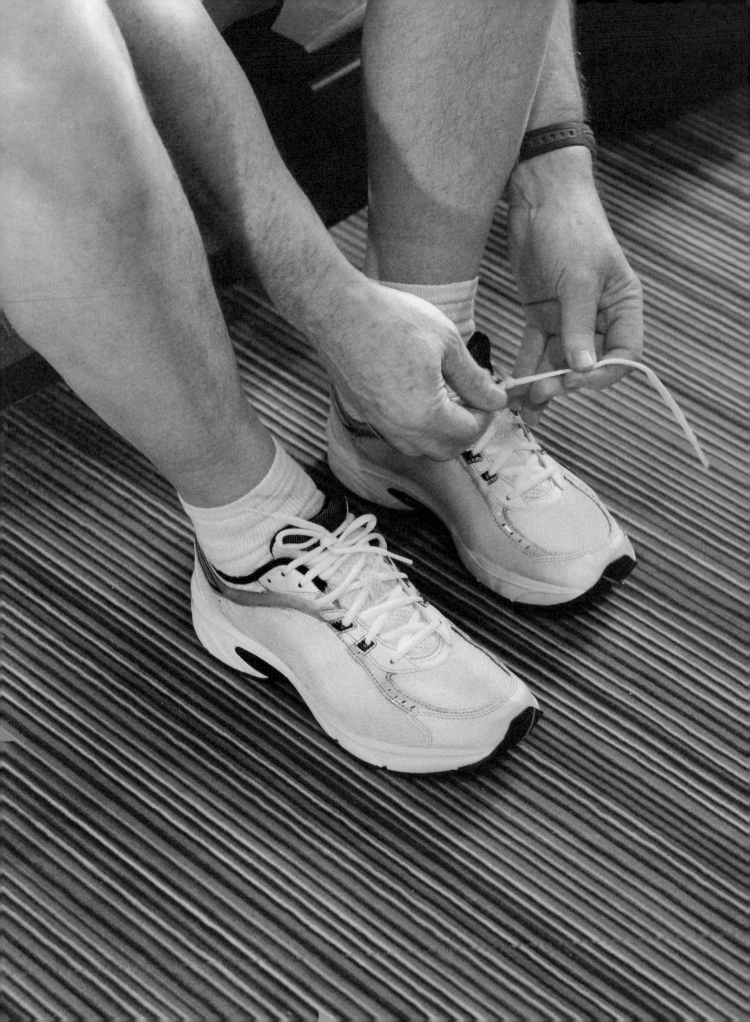

ADDITIONAL MATERIAL

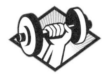

Acknowledgments

❖

Sources

❖

Other Resources

❖

About the Author

❖

Illustrations Credits

Acknowledgments

This book would never, ever have come into being were it not for the core creative team I've long counted on to make me look good. Brigitte LeBlanc's superlative writing skills and sense of flow gave shape to my ideas. As always, the conceptual graphic design and imagery created by Nita Alvarez brought the work to a deeper and more meaningful level. Both have been my valued creative collaborators for more years than we can believe! Thanks also to Connie Broussard, senior designer at the Alvarez Group, for her excellent creative eye and meticulous production work.

This project also benefited greatly from the stellar illustrations of David Preiss, who was a delight to work with and understands what good exercise form is all about; the contributions of Eileen Hansen, a source of athletic inspiration as well as content and resources; and the photographs of Jim Havey of Havey Productions, another longtime collaborator, who captured my Dallas workout as shown in the Epilogue.

Special thanks are due to Mary Norris. Not only did she apply her keen editorial sense to help us strengthen the manuscript, she also found it the perfect home. Her enthusiasm and belief in the project made all the difference. Thank you, Mary!

I am also grateful for the medical expertise lent to our project by Dr. Miriam Morey, who so thoroughly and thoughtfully reviewed the manuscript.

To a large extent, the process of creating this book paralleled and reinforced my own fitness journey. Each was a learning process that enriched the other. Scottie Gassner's training knowledge was indispensable on both scores (although I still refuse to wear any T-shirt proclaiming "Body by Scottie"). So was the kinesiology expertise of Rachel Sosa, who taught me so much about stretching, exercise form, and workout pacing. Then there's Kathleen Crandall, the wonderful yoga, Pilates, and movement teacher who has done so much to help me transform my body, and my life—so long, aches and pains. And let's not forget the gifted hands of Josh Clifton, whose healing massages enabled me to get looser and more flexible than I'd imagined possible. (By the way, Josh, I'm still waiting for my senior discount.)

I cannot say enough to express my gratitude to the immensely talented and professional team at National Geographic Books for their support and wholehearted commitment to the project. I particularly wish to thank Lisa Thomas, senior vice president and editorial director; Susan Straight, senior editorial project manager; and Bill O'Donnell, sales director. At every stage, they have gone above and beyond to ensure the book's quality and success.

Last but not least (unless I want to sleep by myself), I want to thank Stanya, my bride of 48 years, for being by my side at every step of this process and on every one of our walks. Without her patience and unselfishness, this book would not exist.

Sources

CHAPTER 1

AARP Livable Communities. "The United States of Aging Survey—2012." http://www.aarp.org/content/dam/aarp/livable-communities/learn/research/the-united-states-of-aging-survey-2012-aarp.pdf.

American Academy of Orthopaedic Surgeons. "Beyond Surgery Day: The Full Impact of Knee Replacement," *A Nation in Motion,* 2016. http://www.anationinmotion.org/value/knee/.

Arthritis Foundation. "What Is Arthritis?" http://www.arthritis.org/about-arthritis/understanding-arthritis/what-is-arthritis.php.

Babyak, Michael, James A. Blumenthal, Steve Herman, Parinda Khatri, Murali Doraiswamy, Kathleen Moore, W. Edward Craighead, Teri T. Baldewicz, and K. Ranga Krishnan. "Exercise Treatment for Major Depression: Maintenance of Therapeutic Benefit at 10 Months." *Psychosomatic Medicine* 62, no. 5 (2000): 633–8. https://www.madinamerica.com/wp-content/uploads/2011/12/Exercise%20treatment%20for%20major%20depression.pdf.

Berkowitz, Bonnie, and Patterson Clark. "The Health Hazards of Sitting," *Washington Post,* January 20, 2014. https://www.washingtonpost.com/apps/g/page/national/the-health-hazards-of-sitting/750/.

Bergland, Christopher. "The Neurochemicals of Happiness," *The Athlete's Way* (blog), *Psychology Today,* November 29, 2012. https://www.psychologytoday.com/blog/the-athletes-way/201211/the-neurochemicals-happiness.

Bilanow, Toby. "Walking to Age Well," *The New Old Age* (blog), *New York Times,* May 27, 2014. http://newoldage.blogs.nytimes.com/2014/05/27/walking-to-age-well/?_r=0.

Boston Globe. "Long-Term Weight Gain: How Does It Happen?" June 27, 2011. http://archive.boston.com/lifestyle/health/articles/2011/06/27/long_term_weight_gain_how_does_it_happen/.

Brody, Jane E. "Keep Moving to Stay a Step Ahead of Arthritis," *Well* (blog), *New York Times,* April 27, 2015. http://well.blogs.nytimes.com/2015/04/27/keep-moving-even-if-in-new-ways-to-stay-a-step-ahead-of-arthritis/.

Callahan, L. F., J. H. Shreffler, M. Altpeter, B. Schoster, J. Hootman, L. O. Houenou, K. R. Martin, and T. A. Schwartz. "Evaluation of Group and Self-Directed Formats of the Arthritis Foundation's Walk With Ease Program." *Arthritis Care & Research* 63, no. 8 (August 2011): 1098–1107. https://www.ncbi.nlm.nih.gov/pubmed/21560255.

Castillo, Michelle. "Sitting Too Much May Double Your Risk of Dying, Study Shows," CBSNews.com, March 27, 2012. http://www.cbsnews.com/news/sitting-too-much-may-double-your-risk-of-dying-study-shows/.

Coghlan, Andy. "Physical Inactivity Kills as Many People as Smoking," *New Scientist,* July 18, 2012. https://www.newscientist.com/article/dn22072-physical-inactivity-kills-as-many-people-as-smoking/.

DiSalvo, David. "How Exercise Makes Your Brain Grow," *Forbes,* October 13, 2013. http://www.forbes.com/sites/daviddisalvo/2013/10/13/how-exercise-makes-your-brain-grow/#794fa27748c1.

Flegal, Katherine M., Deanna Kruszon-Moran, Margaret D. Carroll, Cheryl D. Fryar, and Cynthia L. Ogden. "Trends in Obesity Among Adults in the United States, 2005 to 2014." *Journal of the American Medication Association* 315, no. 21 (June 7, 2016): 2284–91. http://jamanetwork.com/journals/jama/article-abstract/2526639.

Gardner, Charlie. "Was the Rise of Car Ownership Responsible for the Midcentury Homeownership Boom in the US?" *Old Urbanist* (blog), February 17, 2013. http://oldurbanist.blogspot.com/2013/02/was-rise-of-car-ownership-responsible.html.

Hawkins, Steven A., and Robert A. Wiswell. "Rate and Mechanism of Maximal Oxygen Consumption Decline With Aging." *Sports Medicine* 33, no. 12 (2003): 877–88. http://www.uni.edu/dolgener/cardiovascular_phys/Electronic%20Articles/Maximal_O2_and_Aging.pdf.

Ingraham, Susan. "7 Reasons Older Adults Don't Stay in Exercise Classes," PainScience.com, October 30, 2015. https://www.painscience.com/articles/7-reasons-older-adults-dont-stay-in-exercise-classes.php.

Janot, Jeff M., and Len Kravitz. "Maximizing Functional Abilities in the Older Adult," University of New Mexico, 2000. https://www.unm.edu/~lkravitz/Article%20folder/olderadult.html.

Landa, Jennifer. "How Working Out Can Improve Your Sex Life." *Wellness Watch* (blog), FoxNews.com, September 9, 2013. http://www.foxnews.com/health/2013/09/09/how-working-out-can-improve-your-sex-life/.

Landro, Laura. "Building Better Bones," *Wall Street Journal,* October 25, 2010. http://www.wsj.com/news/articles/SB10001424052748703631704575552632625501358.

LeWine, Howard. "Two-Thirds of Seniors Need Help Doing One or More Daily Activities," *Harvard Health Blog,* December 13, 2013. http://www.health.harvard.edu/blog/two-thirds-of-seniors-need-help-doing-one-or-more-daily-activities-201312136942.

Lewis, Tanya. "Only Half of Americans Got Enough Exercise Last Year—Here's How Much You Should Be Doing," *Business Insider,* February 23, 2016. http://www.businessinsider.com/cdc-report-on-exercise-trends-2016-2.

Marshall, Serena. "Government Sets New Recommended Salt Levels for Foods," ABC7NY.com, June 1, 2016. http://abc7ny.com/news/government-sets-new-recommended-salt-levels-for-foods/1366290/.

Morey, Miriam C., Ph.D. (professor of geriatric medicine, Duke University School of Medicine), in discussion with Brigitte LeBlanc, November 6, 2016.

National Osteoporosis Foundation. "Just for Men," 2016. https://www.nof.org/prevention/general-facts/just-for-men/.

Nelson, Miriam E., W. Jack Rejeski, Steven N. Blair, Pamela W. Duncan, James O. Judge, Abby C. King, Carol A. Macera, and Carmen Castaneda-Sceppa. "Physical Activity and Public Health in Older Adults: Recommendation From the American College of Sports Medicine and the American Heart Association," *Circulation* 116, no. 9 (2007): 1094–1105. http://scholarcommons.sc.edu/sph_epidemiology_biostatistics_facpub/380/.

NIHSeniorHealth. "Falls and Older Adults," October 16, 2006. https://nihseniorhealth.gov/falls/aboutfalls/01.html.

Paris, Valerie. "Why Do Americans Spend So Much on Pharmaceuticals?" *PBS NewsHour*, February 7, 2014. http://www.pbs.org/newshour/updates/americans-spend-much-pharmaceuticals/.

Reynolds, Gretchen. "Ask Well: When Sitting Can Be Good for You," *Well* (blog), *New York Times*, October 9, 2015. http://well.blogs.nytimes.com/2015/10/09/ask-well-when-sitting-can-be-good-for-you/.

——. "Older Athletes Have a Strikingly Young Fitness Age," *Well* (blog), *New York Times*, July 1, 2016. http://well.blogs.nytimes.com/2015/07/01/older-athletes-have-a-strikingly-young-fitness-age/.

——. "What's Your Fitness Age?" *Well* (blog), *New York Times*, October 15, 2014. http://well.blogs.nytimes.com/2014/10/15/whats-your-fitness-age/.

——. "Why Fidgeting Is Good Medicine." *Well* (blog), *New York Times*, September 14, 2016. http://www.nytimes.com/2016/09/14/well/move/why-fidgeting-is-good-medicine.html.

ScienceDaily. "Nearly 7 in 10 Americans Are on Prescription Drugs," June 19, 2013. https://www.sciencedaily.com/releases/2013/06/130619132352.htm.

Servick, Kelly. "How Exercise Beefs Up the Brain," *Science*, October 10, 2013. http://www.sciencemag.org/news/2013/10/how-exercise-beefs-brain.

Shaw, Gina. "Exercise and Pain Relief," WebMD, 2005. http://www.webmd.com/pain-management/features/exercise-relief.

University of California, Davis, Health System. "This Is Your Brain on Exercise," *Newsroom* (blog), February 23, 2016. https://www.ucdmc.ucdavis.edu/publish/news/newsroom/10798.

U.S. Centers for Disease Control and Prevention. "Arthritis-Related Statistics," updated October 5, 2016. http://www.cdc.gov/arthritis/data_statistics/arthritis-related-stats.htm.

——. "Chronic Disease Prevention and Health Promotion," updated August 16, 2016. http://www.cdc.gov/chronicdisease/.

——. "Home and Recreational Safety: Important Facts About Falls," updated September 20, 2016. http://www.cdc.gov/homeandrecreationalsafety/falls/adultfalls.html.

——. "QuickStats: Mean Percentage Body Fat, by Age Group and Sex—National Health and Nutrition Examination Survey, United States, 1999–2004," January 2, 2009. http://www.cdc.gov/mmwr/preview/mmwrhtml/mm5751a4.htm.

Wanlass, Jason. "Take the Path of Most Resistance," *Idaho Statesman*, June 8, 2015. http://www.idahostatesman.com/news/nation-world/health-and-medicine/article40862559.html.

Watkins, James. "Physical Activity Helps Reduce Bone Loss," Human Kinetics, May 12, 2011. http://www.humankinetics.com/excerpts/excerpts/physical-activity-helps-reduce-bone-loss.

CHAPTER 2

Hauser, Annie. "30 Minutes of Exercise Does the Trick, Study Says," EverydayHealth.com, August 24, 2012. http://www.everydayhealth.com/fitness/0824/30-minutes-of-exercise-does-the-trick-study-says.aspx.

Kleiman, Karen. "Try Some Smile Therapy," *This Isn't What I Expected* (blog), *Psychology Today*, August 1, 2012. https://www.psychologytoday.com/blog/isnt-what-i-expected/201207/try-some-smile-therapy.

Peterson, Christopher. "Smiling and Stress," *The Good Life* (blog), *Psychology Today*, September 13, 2012. https://www.psychologytoday.com/blog/the-good-life/201209/smiling-and-stress.

Rubin, Gretchen. *Better Than Before: What I Learned about Making and Breaking Habits—to Sleep More, Quit Sugar, Procrastinate Less, and Generally Build a Happier Life*. United States: Broadway Books, 2015.

Statistic Brain. "New Years Resolution Statistics," accessed November 7, 2016. http://www.statisticbrain.com/new-years-resolution-statistics/.

Torgovnick May, Kate. "Kelly McGonigal on Why It's So Dang Hard to Stick to a Resolution," *TED Blog*, January 8, 2014. http://blog.ted.com/the-science-of-willpower-kelly-mcgonigal-on-why-its-so-dang-hard-to-stick-to-a-resolution/.

Wright, Vonda, and Ruth Winter. *Fitness After 40: How to Stay Strong at Any Age*. New York: AMACOM, 2009.

CHAPTER 3

Browning, Dominique. "I'm Too Old for This," *New York Times*, August 8, 2015. http://www.nytimes.com/2015/08/09/fashion/im-too-old-for-this.html.

Duenwald, Mary. "Power of Positive Thinking Extends, It Seems, to Aging," *New York Times*, November 19, 2002. http://www.nytimes

.com/2002/11/19/science/power-of-positive-thinking-extends-it
-seems-to-aging.html.

Ellin, Abby. "Hitting the Gym and the Trails, Looking to Extend the
Golden Years," *New York Times,* July 31, 2015. http://www.nytimes
.com/2015/08/01/your-money/health-clubs-and-resorts-catch-on
-with-older-adults.html?hpw&rref=business&action=click&pgtype
=Homepage&module=well-region&region=bottom well&WT.nav
=bottom-well.

Godman, Heidi. "Feeling Young at Heart May Help You Live Longer,"
Harvard Health Blog, December 17, 2014. http://www.health
.harvard.edu/blog/feeling-young-heart-may-help-live-longer
-201412177598.

Windhorst, Brian. "LeBron's Extra Edge: Cavaliers Star's Devotion to
Yoga Training Helps Keep James Healthy," *Plain Dealer,* March
23, 2009. http://www.cleveland.com/cavs/index.ssf/2009/03/
lebrons_extra_edge_cavaliers_s.html.

CHAPTER 4

CalorieLab. "Calories Burned by Walking," 2015. http://calorielab
.com/burned/?mo=se&gr=17&ti=walking&q=&wt=150&un=lb
&kg=68.

Cimons, Marlene. "Frailty Is a Medical Condition, Not an Inevitable
Result of Aging," *Washington Post,* December 10, 2012. https://
www.washingtonpost.com/national/health-science/frailty-is-a
-medical-condition-not-an-inevitable-result-of-aging/2012/12/10/
b1cca8a2-f6a7-11e1-8253-3f495ae70650_story.html.

Emilio, Emilio J. Martínez-López, Fidel Hita-Contreras, Pilar M.
Jiménez-Lara, Pedro Latorre-Román, and Antonio Martínez-
Amat. "The Association of Flexibility, Balance, and Lumbar
Strength With Balance Ability: Risk of Falls in Older Adults,"
Journal of Sports Science & Medicine 13, no. 2 (May 2014):
349–57. https://www.ncbi.nlm.nih.gov/pmc/articles/PMC3990
889/.

Fell, James S. "The Myth of Ripped Muscles and Calorie Burns,"
Los Angeles Times, May 16, 2011. http://articles.latimes.com/2011/
may/16/health/la-he-fitness-muscle-myth-20110516.

Fetters, K. Aleisha. "Older Adults: Double Your Protein Intake for
Better Health," *U.S. News & World Report,* February 13, 2015.
http://health.usnews.com/health-news/health-wellness/arti-
cles/2015/02/13/older-adults-double-your-protein-intake-for
-better-health.

Hauser, Annie. "30 Minutes of Exercise Does the Trick, Study Says,"
EverydayHealth.com, August 24, 2012. http://www.everydayhealth
.com/fitness/0824/30-minutes-of-exercise-does-the-trick-study
-says.aspx.

International Osteoporosis Foundation. "Know and Reduce Your Risk
of Osteoporosis," 2007. https://www.iofbonehealth.org/sites/
default/files/PDFs/know_and_reduce_your_risk_english.pdf.

Kadey, Matthew. "The Ultimate List of 40 High-Protein Foods!"
Bodybuilding.com, October 4, 2016. http://www.bodybuilding.
com/content/ultimate-list-40-high-protein-foods.html.

Morey, Miriam C., Ph.D. (professor of geriatric medicine, Duke University School of Medicine), in discussion with Brigitte LeBlanc,
November 6, 2016.

Nelson, Miriam E., W. Jack Rejeski, Steven N. Blair, Pamela W. Duncan,
James O. Judge, Abby C. King, Carol A. Macera, and Carmen
Castaneda-Sceppa. "Physical Activity and Public Health in Older
Adults: Recommendation From the American College of Sports
Medicine and the American Heart Association," *Circulation* 116,
no. 9 (2007): 1094–1105. http://scholarcommons.sc.edu/sph_
epidemiology_biostatistics_facpub/380/.

Metzl, Jordan D., and Andrew Heffernan. *The Exercise Cure: A Doctor's All-Natural, No-Pill Prescription for Better Health & Longer
Life.* New York: Rodale, 2014.

NIHSeniorHealth. "Falls and Older Adults," October 16, 2006. https://
nihseniorhealth.gov/falls/aboutfalls/01.html.

Reynolds, Gretchen. "Aging Well Through Exercise," *Well* (blog),
New York Times, November 9, 2011. http://well.blogs.nytimes
.com/2011/11/09/aging-well-through-exercise/?utm_source=
twitterfeed&utm_medium=twitter&utm_campaign=NYT
+Wellness.

Ullrich, Peter F., Jr. "Exercise and Back Pain," Spine-Health.com,
accessed November 9, 2016. http://www.spine-health.com/
wellness/exercise/exercise-and-back-pain.

University of North Carolina School of Medicine. "Chronic Low Back
Pain on the Rise: UNC Study Finds 'Alarming Increase' in Preva-
lence." February 9, 2009. http://www.med.unc.edu/www/news
archive/2009/february/chronic-low-back-pain-on-the-rise-unc
-study-finds-alarming-increase-in-prevalence.

U.S. Centers for Disease Control and Prevention. "Home and Recreational Safety: Important Facts About Falls," updated September
20, 2016. http://www.cdc.gov/homeandrecreationalsafety/falls/
adultfalls.html.

Vellas, B. J., S. J. Wayne, L. J. Romero, R. N. Baumgartner, and P. J.
Garry. "Fear of Falling and Restriction of Mobility in Elderly Fall-
ers," *Age and Ageing* 26, no. 3 (May 1997): 189–93. https://www
.ncbi.nlm.nih.gov/pubmed/9223714.

Wanlass, Jason. "Take the Path of Most Resistance," *Idaho Statesman,*
June 8, 2015. http://www.idahostatesman.com/news/nation-world/
health-and-medicine/article40862559.html.

Watson, Stephanie. "Try Tai Chi to Improve Balance, Avoid Falls,"
Harvard Health Blog, August 23, 2012. http://www.health.harvard
.edu/blog/try-tai-chi-to-improve-balance-avoid-falls-20120823
5198.

WebMD. "Osteoporosis: Are You at Risk?" October 23, 2016. http://
www.webmd.com/osteoporosis/guide/osteoporosis-risk-factors.

Wright, Vonda, and Ruth Winter. *Fitness After 40: How to Stay Strong at Any Age*. New York: AMACOM, 2009.

CHAPTER 5

Van Pelt, Jennifer. "Exercise as Medicine," *Today's Geriatric Medicine* 3, no. 1 (Winter 2010): 18. http://www.todaysgeriatricmedicine .com/archive/020110p18.shtml.

Wright, Vonda, and Ruth Winter. *Fitness After 40: How to Stay Strong at Any Age*. New York: AMACOM, 2009.

CHAPTER 6

American Heart Association. "Walk, Don't Run, Your Way to a Healthy Heart," updated April 18, 2016. http://www.heart.org/HEARTORG/ HealthyLiving/PhysicalActivity/Walking/Walk-Dont-Run-Your-Way -to-a-Healthy-Heart_UCM_452926_Article.jsp#.VuIX2dAnKMM.

Brody, Jane E. "Posture Affects Standing, and Not Just the Physical Kind," *Well* (blog), *New York Times*, December 28, 2015. http:// well.blogs.nytimes.com/2015/12/28/posture-affects-standing-and -not-just-the-physical-kind/.

Clear, James. "How to Be Confident and Reduce Stress in 2 Minutes per Day," JamesClear.com, July 25, 2013. http://jamesclear.com/ body-language-how-to-be-confident.

Reynolds, Gretchen. "Is It Better to Walk or Run?" *Well* (blog), *New York Times*, May 29, 2013. http://well.blogs.nytimes.com/2013/05/ 29/is-it-better-to-walk-or-run/?_r=0.

U.S. Centers for Disease Control and Prevention. "Physical Activity and Health," updated June 4, 2015. https://www.cdc.gov/physical activity/basics/pa-health/.

CHAPTER 7

Ericson, John. "75% of Americans May Suffer From Chronic Dehydration, According to Doctors," *Medical Daily*, July 3, 2013. http:// www.medicaldaily.com/75-americans-may-suffer-chronic -dehydration-according-doctors-247393.

Mayo Clinic. "Water: How Much Should You Drink Every Day?" September 5, 2014. http://www.mayoclinic.org/healthy-lifestyle/ nutrition-and-healthy-eating/in-depth/water/art-20044256.

McMahon, Gerard E, Christopher I. Morse, Adrian Burden, Keith Winwood, and Gladys L. Onambélé. "Impact of Range of Motion During Ecologically Valid Resistance Training Protocols on Muscle Size, Subcutaneous Fat, and Strength," *Journal of Strength and Conditioning Research* 28, no. 1 (January 2014): 245–55. http:// journals.lww.com/nsca-jscr/Citation/2014/01000/Impact_of_ Range_of_Motion_During_Ecologically.32.aspx.

National Institutes of Health. "Nutrient Recommendations: Dietary Reference Intakes," updated October 17, 2016. https://ods.od.nih .gov/Health_Information/Dietary_Reference_Intakes.aspx.

U.S. Bureau of Labor Statistics. "Occupational Outlook Handbook: Fitness Trainers and Instructors," December 17, 2015. http:// www.bls.gov/ooh/personal-care-and-service/fitness-trainers-and -instructors.htm.

CHAPTER 9

Eat This, Not That. "19 Salads Worse Than a Whopper," January 22, 2016. http://www.eatthis.com/19-salads-worse-than-whopper.

Gillan, Becky. "Top 10 Demographics & Interests Facts About Americans Age 50+," *AARP Notebook* (blog), May 14, 2014. http:// blog.aarp.org/2014/05/14/top-10-demographics-interests-facts -about-americans-age-50/.

Kane, Andrea. "How Fat Affects Arthritis," ArthritisFoundation.com, 2016. http://www.arthritis.org/living-with-arthritis/comorbidities/ obesity-arthritis/fat-and-arthritis.php.

National Council on Aging. "Healthy Aging Facts," June 3, 2015. https://www.ncoa.org/news/resources-for-reporters/get-the-facts/ healthy-aging-facts/.

Pew Research Center. "Baby Boomers Retire," December 29, 2010. http://www.pewresearch.org/daily-number/baby-boomers-retire/.

Pollan, Michael. *Food Rules: An Eater's Manual*. New York: Penguin Press, 2009.

Reynolds, Gretchen. "Ask Well: When Sitting Can Be Good for You," *Well* (blog), *New York Times*, October 9, 2015. http://well.blogs .nytimes.com/2015/10/09/ask-well-when-sitting-can-be-good -for-you/.

———. "Is It Better to Walk or Run?" *Well* (blog), *New York Times*, May 29, 2013. http://well.blogs.nytimes.com/2013/05/29/is-it-better-to -walk-or-run/?_r=0.

U.S. Census Bureau. "Fueled by Aging Baby Boomers, Nation's Older Population to Nearly Double in the Next 20 Years, Census Bureau Reports," May 6, 2014. http://www.census.gov/newsroom/press -releases/2014/cb14-84.html.

U.S. News & World Report. "*U.S. News & World Report* Reveals the 2016 Best Diets Rankings," January 5, 2016. http://www.usnews .com/info/blogs/press-room/2016/01/05/us-news-reveals-the -2016-best-diets-rankings.

Other Resources

If you want to learn more about body mechanics and fitness, here are some places to start.

New York Times Health Section / Well Blog

The *NYT* is my top go-to source for the latest news about health and fitness. The health columns in the *Times's* weekly Science section and the *Well* blog in the online edition are a trove of useful information. I especially enjoy the articles by Jane Brody, the grande dame of personal health reporting, who is now over 75 herself, and her younger colleague, Gretchen Reynolds.

Wall Street Journal

"What's Your Workout?," a regular feature of the *WSJ's* Personal Journal section, lets you peek inside the fitness strategies of top executives and entrepreneurs. Their enthusiasm, and the ways they work fitness into their lives, are always interesting and sometimes inspirational.

Men's Fitness / Men's Health

These magazines are clearly geared to a younger demographic than mine, and plenty of bulging muscles are on display. But amid the lifestyle articles you'll find plenty of good functional exercises and practical workout tips. The same goes for the women's versions. The online editions include videos that illuminate proper form.

The Book of Body Maintenance and Repair
by the American Physical Therapy Association

A terrific all-around reference from the nation's largest association of physical therapist professionals, this book discusses the care and treatment of each body part in direct, straight-to-the-point style. It also provides general information on fitness and an extensive compendium of stretches and exercises.

The Men's Health Big Book of Exercises
The Women's Health Big Book of Exercises
by Adam Campbell

Are exercises for men different from those for women? Not really. But it doesn't matter if the distinction is mainly for marketing purposes. These books are exactly what they promise to be—nicely illustrated, well-organized exercise encyclopedias with excellent notes on form. Workouts geared to different objectives are included.

The Exercise Cure
by Jordan Metzl, M.D.

"Exercise is medicine," says Dr. Jordan Metzl, an M.D. and veteran of many marathons and Ironman challenges. His book translates that philosophy into practical terms with a problem/solution format covering a broad spectrum of conditions and ailments, including a special section on cancer. He provides just enough medical background to explain what's causing symptoms and how exercise can help.

Younger Next Year
by Chris Crowley and Henry S. Lodge, M.D.

This book is the flagship in a series providing plenty of evidence that exercise can lower your biological age. The books are also chock full of commonsense strategies for doing just that, all wrapped in rollicking prose and personal anecdotes. The road to "aha" moments is sometimes long and winding, but it's a pleasant excursion.

go4life.nia.nih.gov

This website from the National Institute on Aging is one of the world's largest and best sources of senior-focused fitness information—and it's all free! They will even send you DVDs and booklets on request.

About the Author

After a successful 35-year Wall Street career, Jim Owen found new purpose in being an author, inspirational speaker, and social entrepreneur. His previous books include *Cowboy Ethics* (2004), a best seller with more than 150,000 copies sold to date, *Cowboy Values* (2008), and *The Try* (2013).

The **Just Move!** initiative is the most recent project of the Center for Cowboy Ethics and Leadership, the nonprofit, 501(c)(3) corporation Jim founded in 2006. At the heart of the center's work is the idea that simple, timeless values and personal character are the keys to tackling some of society's toughest issues. The iconic figure of the American cowboy, who lives by time-honored principles of courage, optimism, and hard work, is emblematic of this philosophy.

The center's mission is to inspire people of all ages to reach for the best in themselves so they can reach their full potential. It presently focuses on three programs:

BE SOMEBODY! is all about young people, our leaders of tomorrow. In these challenging times, it takes something special to succeed in a career, and in life. Through its partnership with the Cherry Creek School District in Denver and the Boys & Girls Clubs of Central Wyoming, the center is helping middle- and high-school-age students develop a strong sense of who they are and what kind of life they want to have. The project has translated the messages of Jim's books into curriculum materials and a training program for teachers and youth-group leaders. To date, the program has trained more than 500 instructors, involved 175 different organizations, and brought inspiration to thousands of young people across at least 20 states.

STANDING TALL! spotlights the issue of business ethics in an era when many Americans feel that large corporations can't be trusted. In a June 2016 Gallup poll, 36 percent of respondents said they had "very little" trust in big business, the highest percentage since 2009, and only 18 percent expressed "a great deal" or "quite a lot" of trust. The center's Standing Tall! workshops are interactive, introspective sessions that help businesspeople define "a code of their own," the principles they want to stand for both inside and outside the workplace. More than 200 workshops have been held around the U.S. thus far, with participants hailing from all 50 states and more than 20 countries. In follow-up surveys, 98 percent of workshop graduates say the experience was "meaningful," and 99 percent of those who created a personal code say it has helped them deal with real-life situations.

JUST MOVE! takes aim at an unfolding crisis affecting a different demographic, the baby boomers who are now moving into retirement. The last of the baby boomer generation turned 50 in 2014, and about 100 million Americans are now 50 or over. Americans are reaching the traditional retirement age of 65 at the rate of 10,000 a day, and our population's share of older people is expected to nearly double by 2030, rising from 12 percent to almost 20 percent.

What makes this a looming crisis is the fact that an estimated 92 percent of older adults have at least one chronic disease, according to the National Council on Aging, and 77 percent have at least two. Shockingly, one out of five current Medicare beneficiaries has five or more chronic conditions! So it's no surprise that chronic diseases account for three-fourths of all U.S. health care spending, and the "big four"—heart disease, cancer, stroke, and diabetes—cause almost two-thirds of all deaths in our country each year.

When Jim reached 70, he realized that many older Americans were in the same boat he was in—out of shape and in danger of watching their mobility and quality of life go down the drain. "The complex health care needs of older Americans are growing at a much faster rate than the resources available to treat them," Jim observes. "At the same time, experts tell us that most of our annual health care spending is directed at conditions that are partly or mostly due to lifestyle choices. Creating a culture of fitness that includes older people, who often assume it's too late for them to get in shape, **has** to be part of the answer."

Jim's search for his own path to fitness led him to write the guide he wished he'd had at the outset. Today he is over 75, in the best shape of his life, and eager to share the secrets of his success. This book and an emerging slate of related activities are the result.

While Jim's newfound passion for fitness may seem like a departure from the center's other programs, the **Just Move!** project reflects many of the same themes that have animated Jim's work for more than a decade—namely, how commitment, focus, and determination can help us reach our goals; the idea that "winning at life" is more important to our happiness than material success; and the responsibility we each hold for shaping our own lives.

"Each of us is the author of our own life story," says Jim, "and if we can stay physically fit, mobile, and independent into old age, the last chapters can be the most rewarding and fulfilling of all."

We can all be heroes in our own lives.
from *Cowboy Ethics*

All it takes... is all you've got.
from *The Try*

Self-reliance grows from taking responsibility for our own well-being.
from *Cowboy Values*

Illustrations Credits

All graphics by Connie Broussard, The Alvarez Group; original art by David Priess.